Mastering the Art of Patient Care

Michelle Kittleson

Mastering the Art of Patient Care

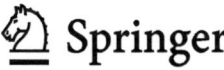 Springer

Michelle Kittleson
Smidt Heart Institute
Cedars-Sinai Medical Center
Los Angeles, CA, USA

ISBN 978-3-031-20919-2   ISBN 978-3-031-20920-8   (eBook)
https://doi.org/10.1007/978-3-031-20920-8

This Springer imprint is published by the registered company Springer Nature Switzerland AG
The registered company address is: Gewerbestrasse 11, 6330 Cham, Switzerland

For my family

Foreword

It has been more years than I would like to admit since I began my journey as a doctor. However, the challenges, uncertainties, and fears of the early days of my training remain indelible in my memory. I cannot help but think how much better off I may have been if "Mastering the Art of Patient Care" had been available to me then.

Being a physician is indeed as much an art as it is a science—something that is easily lost in the whirlwind of back-to-back rotations, late nights on call, and trial-by-fire differentials. Infused with levelheaded logic, an empathetic sensibility, and hard-won wisdom, "Mastering the Art of Patient Care" is a lifeline to those who aspire not only to a successful career, but also to a purpose-filled life in medicine.

Michelle Kittleson has found a way to celebrate preparation, practice (practice, practice), and intellectual curiosity as the cornerstone of professional development; her passion for medicine is evident in every real-world illustration of learning concepts. Insights she gained from mentors who often came in unexpected forms speaks to her expansive understanding of what it means to be a good physician.

Marrying common sense, humor, and practical strategies, Dr. Kittleson offers a model to navigate the complexities of patient care that is inclusive of multidisciplinary collaboration and respect for the patient perspective. She extends the Golden Rule of "do no harm" to embrace the idea that sometimes the best course is doing nothing, and that action should only be taken if it helps the patient feel better and/or live longer. In the process, she reminds us that medicine is a team sport and that every day provides opportunities to learn and grow.

This book is an opening statement, not the concluding remarks of an ongoing conversation in medicine that we should not shy away from having. What is the best way to educate and train the next generation of physicians? How do we support ongoing development so that trainees evolve into knowledgeable professionals with the competency to make decisions under duress as well as compassionate care-givers who find joy in their work? How do we make space for both women and men to integrate family life and other passions into a medical career? How can we better prioritize mentorship of young physicians on processing grief, overcoming the sting of mistakes, and setting boundaries to preserve their own well-being? Michelle

Kittleson has done us all a service by raising these questions and offering her unique viewpoint on answering them.

Over many years, I have seen tremendous growth in this field and many young physicians engaged in the care of these patients. I have seen these physicians take great strides to advance the science of medicine in our field. Among the many outstanding young physicians that I have observed and one who has exceeded all my expectations is Dr. Michelle Kittleson. Rarely do I find someone who is so aware and observant to be able to understand what makes an outstanding physician who can provide outstanding patient care. Having worked shoulder to shoulder with her for more than 15 years, I can attest that she knows of what she speaks and that she practices what she preaches.

From newly minted medical students, established physicians and all of those in between, we would all do well to follow her lead.

Jon A. Kobashigawa, MD

DSL/ Thomas D. Gordon
Professor of Medicine
Director, Advanced Heart Disease Division
Director, Heart Transplant Program
Associate Director, Smidt Heart Institute
Associate Director, Comprehensive Transplant Center
Smidt Heart Institute, Cedars-Sinai Medical Center
Los Angeles, CA, USA

Preface

I am the fifth generation of physicians in my family and an only child. I was told, for as long as I can remember, that I would be a physician. My maternal grandfather was the dean of St. John's Medical College in Bengaluru, India, which is where my parents first met. They studied together for every test, competing for the highest scores. When I went to India as a teenager for the 25th anniversary celebration of St. John's, my family and I walked down the hallways of the medical school, past plaques listing the highest-scoring students by year in anatomy, physiology, biochemistry, microbiology, and so on. Almost without exception, as I recall it, the highest scorers in each subject for the class of 1971 belonged to one of my parents. Soon after medical school graduation, my mom and dad married and moved to the U.S. to start their residencies in pathology and internal medicine, respectively.

As Indian immigrants, they were tiger parents before the term was coined. They may have even been the original tiger parents; who knows? As a mom of three boys, I strive to instill the same values: initiative, pride in one's work, resilience, and determination. I am probably more of a kitten than a tiger, though my small and retractable claws are still pretty sharp.

As early as second grade, my parents and I had exhaustive discussions about who the smartest kid in class was, and what made them so successful. The preparation gathered momentum from there: an "A" on a test was never enough unless it was the highest score in the class. I learned French and piano (which stuck) and tennis (which didn't). Like every kid, I entertained my own fantasy careers: from hairdresser to chef to writer. All the same, I always knew I would be a doctor because that was what my parents told me I would become. I studied hard and amassed the appropriate accolades: captain of the math team, high school valedictorian, stratospheric scores on the medical college admissions test (MCAT), and graduation from college a year early thanks to advanced placement courses in high school. I received acceptance letters from nearly every medical school I applied to.

It came as a surprise to me, then, on the first day of medical school, that my excitement was tinged with real anxiety: the stakes were no longer bragging rights for the highest test score; the stakes were life and death. There was still so much to learn—how would I ever know all of it? I grew up in awe of my parents who could diagnose strangers in restaurants or shopping malls with strokes or emphysema or Parkinson's disease. As the years of medical school went by, I too learned to observe the hemiparesis, pursed-lip breathing, and pill-rolling tremors and intuit the underlying cause. Still, I wasn't practicing medicine for long before I realized that while acquiring medical knowledge is necessary, it is not sufficient for becoming an outstanding physician.

With dedication and determination, nearly anyone can learn physiology and clinical manifestations of cerebrovascular disease, obstructive lung disease, and movement disorders. These subjects are skillfully taught in medical school and, with enough time and effort, are straightforward to master. How do we learn what isn't taught? Explaining long-term care options to a family after their mother has suffered a major stroke, tailoring the approach of smoking cessation counseling to the patient (will exhortation or cajoling work best?), and breaking the news of a progressive neurologic disorder to a devastated new father—that's the real challenge of medicine, and should be its greatest reward. These skills are the other half of being an outstanding physician, yet they are not part of the medical school curriculum.

A love of people and a love of science barely capture the essence of a life in medicine; there is so much more to being a physician than understanding pathophysiology and identifying the most obscure item on the differential diagnosis. Dinnertime conversations with my parents focused on the finer points of pathology and cardiology were meant to prime me for the challenges of medical school. They did—to a degree—but I have made plenty of mistakes along the way. Ask any experienced physician: they will remember all the gory details of their few painful failures much more clearly than those of their many successes.

Some mistakes were minor, like the time a senior surgical resident explained the role of decubitus films in the assessment of pleural effusions, and I asked how chest x-rays could diagnose decubitus ulcers. Other mistakes were more significant and hurt more than my pride. I had observed my attending physicians deliver bad news both skillfully and clumsily; applying their lessons when I had to share bad news for the first time was harder than it looked. Lacking explicit instruction or preparation—never mind a system—I was hesitant, disorganized, and scared. The first time a frustrated patient yelled at me because I did not sufficiently prepare them for the pain of suture removal as I should have, I exited, mid-suture removal, in tears.

I was learning a hard lesson: none of my academic accomplishments had prepared me for mastering the art of patient care. So much effort was spent in medical school on the Krebs cycle and the brachial plexus; why was there so little focus on systematically honing bedside manner? I soon discovered that it would take time and observation and instruction—in a word, experience—to learn to approach suffering and grief and anger with kindness and calm. It would take the same experience to share the joys of the miracles and triumphs of medicine with patients.

Medical knowledge is critical for saving lives yet almost useless without competent bedside manner. Over time, I learned how to listen and break bad news with compassion and gently guide patients through uncomfortable procedures. I learned these lessons through experience, and I owe much of my experience to my mentors. The aphorism goes, "Good judgment comes from experience and experience comes from bad judgment." Where does the bad judgment come from? It comes from inexperience. Does this inexperience always have to be yours? Does it always have to be painful? My answer is no—we can do better—we only need to share what we have learned from our mentors.

The best mentors share their own hard-earned experiences and their bad judgment to help their trainees avoid the same pitfalls. I once asked a mentor, an international expert in heart transplantation, why we were not considering re-transplantation for a patient with cardiogenic shock from rejection maintained on extracorporeal membrane oxygenation support. His response was, "We used to do that, but it didn't work." He went on to explain that in his experience of a handful of cases, most patients who underwent re-transplantation for acute rejection died. Years later, multicenter registry analyses confirmed his observation. With a slight smile, a small shake of his head, and nine words, he epitomized the most important qualities in a mentor: honesty, self-awareness, and humility. Eleanor Roosevelt once said, "Learn from the mistakes of others. You can't live long enough to make them all yourself." Learning from the mistakes of your mentors will provide the most efficient and least painful way for you to gain valuable experience as a fledgling physician. Making mistakes in medicine vicariously is infinitely preferable to making them in reality.

The mentors whom I valued the most would share quick pearls of wisdom on rounds, distilled from their bad judgment. As I gained experience, I amassed pearls of my own, and would jokingly refer to every piece of advice on rounds as "Kittleson Rule Number 1." A particularly dedicated fellow collected about 30 of my rules and emailed them to me after graduation. I shared the email with a few colleagues and every so often, a printout would surface among trainees.

That was as far as it went until the Fall of 2018 when another fellow asked, "Why aren't these pearls on Twitter?" I frowned, telling him that technology in general, and social media in particular, wasn't for me; I still harbor a suspicion for fax machines. As a medical student in the late 1990s, I would call the nearby hospital after I had faxed the patient's release of medical information form. I could never quite believe that the piece of paper I fed through the machine could appear in a medical records department, miles away, over a telephone line. Every time an administrator confirmed receipt of the form, I was amazed that it had worked. And social media took technology to another level: all the sharing (oversharing?)! Did anyone really care what I ate for breakfast? (I later learned that, of course, breakfast selfies were more appropriate for Instagram—which I don't even know how to use).

Luckily, my Twitter-savvy fellow soon changed my mind, bringing up timely studies on rounds. When I asked how he knew more about late-breaking trials than I did, he showed me lively discussion threads attempting to analyze the finer points—from Twitter. I was impressed and humbled and knew better than to dismiss his advice. While he might have been inexperienced in medicine, he understood far more than I did about social media. My mentee became my mentor; he set up my Twitter account.

I soon realized the power of Twitter: while pontificating to the captive audience of 4-6 rotating residents and fellows on rounds, I could also reach an ever-expanding audience of like-minded individuals passionate about medical education and patient care. By April 2019, #kittlesonrules was born, a compendium of random thoughts on how to improve patient care from the nuts-and-bolts of heart failure management to optimizing communication with patients and colleagues to learning from mistakes.

I envisioned #kittlesonrules like a desk calendar, where instead of encountering a little joke or inspirational quotation, each day would start with a useful medical lesson. Of course, explaining the nuances of optimal patient care requires more than 240 characters. I wanted to transform #kittlesonrules into a handbook for those struggling as I did with the unique and overwhelming challenges of medical school and beyond.

The art of patient care is an apprenticeship guided by the wisdom of mentors. I was lucky to have found mine. Propinquity matters, as does compatibility, being open to possibility, and chance. The support you receive and the epiphanies you experience shouldn't come down to random luck. If we amass this accumulated wisdom, we can help future generations experience the joy of medicine as they gain experience with more support and encouragement and less fear and uncertainty than we have endured.

I worked with a cardiothoracic surgeon renowned for his technical skills. As the legend goes, assistants in the operating room would stay out of the surgical field because his hands moved so fast: they were afraid their gloves would be sutured to an anastomosis if they lingered too long. His patients had the shortest duration of cardiopulmonary bypass time and exited the operating room on minimal amounts of inotropic support. I knew early on that I did not have the temperament of a surgeon: the endless hours of dissection coupled with moments of sheer panic did not appeal to me. Still, I was curious: what did a legendary surgeon do in the midst of life-and-death chaos? I encountered him walking down the hall one day and asked. He told me it was simple: when faced with a crashing patient, he enacted a list that he had honed through years of experience, now almost unconsciously, running through the possibilities of why the patient was crashing and what he could do to fix it. He was brilliant; he also had a system. It's been my experience that all great physicians I admire have a system.

Medical training is all-consuming and at times demoralizing; this handbook is my contribution toward making it better. This handbook is my system of surviving and thriving in medicine. It is not the only system but I hope it will be the start of a discussion among physicians to make medical education better. I hope you will integrate my advice with the many lessons you take away from your mentors and patients to fashion your successful styles of practice. Even better, I hope you share the wisdom you have learned to perpetuate a legacy of shared wisdom and apprenticeship in medical education. Together, we can perpetuate the art of medicine.

While nothing can fully prepare you for the fear and anxiety that comes with inexperience, this book can ease some of that uncertainty. Like a mentor, you may turn to in times of crisis, here you will find the wisdom I have gained from my countless mentors and patients. I hope that sharing my successes and failures inspires you to share yours, and helps you thrive as a physician who takes outstanding care of patients, colleagues, and trainees and derive great joy from saving lives.

Los Angeles, USA   Michelle Kittleson

Acknowledgments

The idea for this book began (where else?) on Twitter. Dr. Mark Reid, author of *Medical Axioms*, noticed my early tweets and sent me a copy of his book as inspiration. The lively discourse on #medtwitter—too many wonderful people to name, but you know who you are—spurred me onward. Dr. James Januzzi advised me to write a book of #kittlesonrules before someone else did, and then connected me with Grant Weston, his editor at Springer.

Once the draft was written, my extraordinary husband read through 11 (that's right, eleven) revisions. Unlike the infamous Reviewer 2 well-known to anyone who's ever submitted a manuscript to a scientific journal, my husband's feedback was a perfect balance of encouragement and constructive criticism. I am also thankful for my superb beta-readers, Blake Lindsley and Bret Easton Ellis—not only for their wisdom, but also for their friendship.

I am indebted to my many, many mentors. Their wisdom shines on every page of the book. Without their patience and generosity, I would not be able to guide others to experience the joys of medicine.

Most of all, I am grateful to countless patients and their families, those people who have astounded me with their grace, optimism, strength, and kindness in the face of adversity. I am humbled that they have placed their trust and their lives in my hands. Without them, this book would not be possible.

Contents

About the Author

Michelle Kittleson is the Director of Education in Heart Failure and Transplantation and Professor of Medicine at the Smidt Heart Institute, Cedars-Sinai. She graduated from Harvard College and received her medical degree from Yale University. She completed her residency at Brigham and Women's Hospital and a cardiology fellowship at Johns Hopkins, where she also received a PhD in Clinical Investigation.

Dr. Kittleson is the Deputy Editor of the *Journal of Heart and Lung Transplantation*, on Guideline Writing Committees for the American College of Cardiology/American Heart Association, Co-Editor-in-Chief for the American College of Cardiology Heart Failure Self-Assessment Program, and on the Board of Directors for the Heart Failure Society of America. Her essays have appeared in *New England Journal of Medicine*, *Annals of Internal Medicine*, and *JAMA Cardiology* and her poems have been published in *JAMA* and *Annals of Internal Medicine*.

She has been the recipient of numerous awards and honors, including the Samuel A. Levine Young Clinical Investigator Award from the American Heart Association, Clinical Faculty Teaching Award from the UCLA Department of Medicine, and the Jon A. Kobashigawa Faculty Teaching Award at Cedars-Sinai.

Part I
Building Your Medical Foundation

Chapter 1
Medical School

1.1 The Early Years

I meet lots of wide-eyed college graduates on their way to medical school and I'm often asked what advice I would give. Here are the answers to the universal questions hundreds of students have asked me over the years. Being never shy and always generous with advice, whether solicited or unsolicited, I tell them that the first two years of medical school are not any harder than college. In fact, the first two years of medical school, with all the classes and textbooks, are just an extension of college. This can be disappointing because you cannot wait to do all the things that a real doctor can do. Still, accept that the first two years are necessary and, for the most part, will not be as exciting as you imagined—reality never is.

Medical school is about learning a foreign language and on the most fundamental level, vocabulary and grammar cannot be reasoned out; they must be memorized. Though I was as discouraged as everyone else was with the drudgery of those early years, I thought back to other times in my life when I had to learn a new skill and remembered the moments when my efforts were finally rewarded. One formative experience where I experienced the joyous transformation from drudgery to understanding was learning to speak French.

When I was seven years old, my parents took a vacation to Paris. They returned, enamored by the culture, the food, the history, and most of all by the language. Incandescent with ambition, they subsequently concluded, naturally, that their seven-year-old daughter should learn French. For most parents, this might result in a mental note to sign their kid up for French class in middle school. Not my parents! No, my parents took it upon themselves to find a friend of a friend who taught French at a local college and ask her to tutor me on Saturday mornings. I was thrilled by this turn of events; I adored the *Madeline* stories (Bemelmans 1963). The eponymous heroine was also seven years old, yet so exotic with her bright red hair and Parisian adventures. I expected to learn French by osmosis; a few quick lessons and I'd be ready for summers in Paris, eating *pain au chocolat* with my new best French friend (who would be named Madeline, of course).

© The Author(s), under exclusive license to Springer Nature Switzerland AG 2022   3
M. Kittleson, *Mastering the Art of Patient Care*,
https://doi.org/10.1007/978-3-031-20920-8_1

My parents' request, that a college professor tutor their young daughter, was initially met with amusement and perhaps faint horror, though my parents have never let minor inconveniences like that stop them. Soon they were dropping me off at her home every Saturday morning for an hour. She was so elegant, dark hair in a French pixie cut (it might not have been French, per se, but to an impressionable 7-year-old, it seemed so *French*) and immaculate polished nails, always bluntly cut, rounded, and the most *French* shade of red. We would work in her attic office, at the drafting table she used for a desk. The desk stood atop a zebra rug she had acquired on a safari in Africa (this was the 1980s, when such things were not yet verboten).

The lessons were filled with memorization: masculine and feminine nouns, conjugating verbs, remembering tenses. The first time I realized that all the memorization was actually good for something occurred when we read Le Pont Mirabeau by Guillaume Apollinaire: *"Sous le pont Mirabeau coule la Seine/Et nos amours/Faut-il qu'il m'en souvienne/La joie venait toujours après la peine."* ["Under the Mirabeau bridge/Flows the Seine/And our loves/I must remember them/Joy always followed pain."] Though I stumbled over the words, I felt the beauty of the poem. Instead of automatically translating the French into English in my head, I was able to appreciate the beauty in the sounds and rhythms of the language.

Years later, I did spend a week in the outskirts of Paris with my French pen pal, chatting easily with the shopkeepers as we purchased *pate de campagne* and *bleu d'Auvergne* for a picnic, and I wasn't even disappointed that she wasn't named Madeline.

The slow, plodding process of medical school will be filled with epiphanies like this, borne of thankless drudgery. You will spend hours memorizing the mechanisms of action, indications, contraindications, and side effects of every prescription medication ever approved by the Food and Drug Administration, and it will feel like punishment. Yet a few years later, you'll be caring for patients on clinical rotations and there will come a moment when someone suggests ordering haloperidol to treat delirium in a patient with Parkinson's disease. You'll remember that haloperidol, by blocking dopamine receptors, is contraindicated in patients with Parkinson's disease. This fundamental knowledge base is essential and half of being an outstanding physician.

The hours you spend in the medical library will pay off. Your foundation of medical knowledge, the grammar and vocabulary, will create the most beautiful poetry of all—the poetry of providing optimal patient care. To sustain yourself through the overwhelming deluge of information of the first years of medical school, look back on the times in your life when the plodding effort of learning a new skill finally paid off. Just like that, in medical school, there will be flashes of real inspiration that make the drudgery worthwhile.

Anatomy, physiology, pharmacology, microbiology are just like a foreign language: half the struggle is learning what all the new words mean. My medical school roommates and I would sit around the dining table and practice pronouncing words like norepinephrine and adductor longus. To this day, I do this with new drugs, though levetiracetam and daratumumab still make me stumble.

So how do you thrive in the first two years of medicine? You memorize, memorize, memorize. Memorization is the gateway to knowledge. Find a system that works and stick with it. My system was active, rather than passive, learning. My two active means of learning were: (1) copying cheat sheets; and (2) answering study questions.

1.1.1   The Cheat-Sheet Method

I envied friends with photographic memories. I wish I had it so easy: I could never just allow the information from lectures or textbooks to wash over me and be magically absorbed. I couldn't highlight a page and then know it forever. I had to read the text, listen to the lecture, and then write out a cheat sheet of all the important information. This could mean the mechanism of action, indications, and side effects for cephalosporins, or the brachial plexus anatomy and lesions. Something magical happens when you write something down repeatedly: you never forget it.

Once I had created a high-yield cheat sheet, I would then copy it over and over again, ever condensing and consolidating the information on the page and, by extension, into my brain. This took days, weeks, and months in the medical school library. The time and effort were worth it: it's hard to daydream when you're actively summarizing and copying information repeatedly. The information becomes second-nature. Even more important, this active learning replaces rumination and despair (How will I ever learn all of this? What am I going to do?) with a concrete action plan. You can't worry when you're actively taking steps to accomplish your goals.

1.1.2   Study Questions

There is no better way to learn something than to answer a question about it. For this purpose, books and books of study questions exist. I would use these quiz questions and I would also write my own. Writing flash cards with quiz questions helped me identify and emphasize high-yield material and became a useful tool for study partners too. For example: what is the lesion in the brachial plexus responsible for Erb's palsy and how does it manifest on examination; or list the third-generation cephalosporins and the organisms they target.

1.1.3   Keep Hope Alive

The essential memorization can be dreary and monotonous. There are flashes of utility: at least I'll know to prescribe ceftazidime and not cephalexin if I ever encounter a patient with Pseudomonas pneumonia. Still, for the most part, the knowledge exists in the ether, untethered to any practical use. It will be years before you are on clinical rotations and can apply your knowledge to save lives. How to keep hope alive? For me, inspiration came in the form of television medical dramas and medical memoirs.

ER, the NBC powerhouse, premiered in September 1994; I started medical school in September 1995 when John Carter joined the cast as the wide-eyed, fumbling, and caring medical student in the ER. I felt as if we learned and grew together. Improbably, this television drama maintained my faith that the dreary monotony of the first two years of medical school would end in dramatic saves and lasting bonds with patients and colleagues. (Have no fear: if you're in need of a medical drama to sustain your faith in medical training, you can stream episodes of ER on Hulu.).

In addition to the classic medical TV drama, medical memoirs also sustained me. *The Spirit Catches You and You Fall Down*, by Anne Fadiman is an anthropologic treatise on the gap between a Hmong patient, her family, and her American physicians (Fadiman 1997). As a third year medical student, I borrowed my roommate's copy and it kept me awake for nights. I absorbed the details of how to employ the triangular seating arrangement of interpreter, patient, and physician, always speaking directly to the patient and observing the patient's reactions as the interpreter relays the messages. *The Spirit Catches You and You Fall Down* was a cautionary tale about the dangers of miscommunication. I resolved that, armed with the knowledge from this book, I would do better.

The other book that sustained me through medical school was *My Own Country*, by Abraham Verghese (Verghese 1995). The tale of a displaced Indian physician in the wilds of eastern Tennessee during the AIDS epidemic of the 1980s is an amazing tale of bridging cultures, from Indian to American, from urban to rural, from hetero- to homosexual, from accepted to disenfranchised. *My Own Country* was a window into my future in medicine. Like the author, I longed to have close connections with patients. I could not wait to be a part of their lives, through the joys and the tragedies. Reading *My Own Country*, I could envision a time when all the medical knowledge I was accumulating would have purpose and I would be a real doctor.

Not everyone loves television dramas and medical memoirs as much as I do. For one of my co-residents, the light at the end of the seemingly thankless tunnel of didactic medical education was to channel his obsession with the statistics of professional basketball players into memorizing medical facts, and it worked. He used the same commitment he once devoted to knowing every player's free throw percentages and blocked shots into the drug–drug interactions of the cytochrome P450 system. For another colleague, it was memories of her shifts as an emergency medical technician in college that sustained her. She knew how it felt to have useful and practical knowledge that saved lives. When the memorization became too much, she would remember the rewards. Whatever the strategy, trainees must find their focus.

The stakes are high in medicine. Failing at a French lesson might later earn you an eyeroll from a Parisian waiter. Missing a note at a piano recital might make you cringe with embarrassment, though you can redeem your reputation if you execute the rest of the piece flawlessly. Medical mistakes cost you more than your pride. Neglecting the knowledge that is the foundation of medical care will endanger countless lives.

You may maintain your light at the end of the memorization tunnel by remembering the transformations of unintelligible sounds into the beauty of French poetry or through the inspiration of television dramas, medical memoirs, or prior experiences in patient care. However you keep hope alive, remember the importance of a foundation. Scales before arpeggios, follow the recipe before you create your own—with patience and dedication to the vocabulary and grammar of medicine, you will soon be able to appreciate its poetry.

1.2 The Clinical Years

There are three tough transitions in a physician's career: the transition from the didactic to the clinical years of medical school, from first-year to second-year resident, and from trainee to attending physician (more on tough transitions in Chap. 8). Each transition requires new skills that must be mastered though they are never explicitly taught. My goal is to provide you with a system so that you will thrive during the clinical years of medical school. Of course, this is not the only system—it's the system that I established through my experience and that of my mentors. You will establish your own style. Consider this just the advice of another mentor, one approach to add to your vicarious experience armamentarium.

I'm sometimes asked how much money it would take to make me repeat medical school. Before kids, I would have said no sum was worth the agony of an uncertain future. After kids, I can provide a sum, astounding in both its size and exactitude, encompassing the costs of education, mortgage, and nursing home care. The point is, medical school is hard. The first two years are arduous though by this stage in your education, you know what to do: study a lot and keep up with the assignments, and you will succeed.

The second two years of medical school are more challenging because the rules are different. Evaluations are subjective, and the criteria upon which you are judged are unspoken and subtly change with every rotation. Where to sit, where to stand, when to sit, when to stand, when to speak, when not to speak, what to say, where's the closest bathroom... every decision point comes with a chance of a *faux-pas* (e.g., the time I was hanging on my attending physician's words so closely that I followed her into the restroom. She smiled and politely told me that it would be fine to wait outside). Evaluations are based on the smallest of impressions and medical students feel superfluous and almost always in the way.

My first rotation as a third-year medical student was in cardiothoracic surgery. The clerkship administrator told me that rounds started at 6 AM in the cardiothoracic surgical intensive care unit and I laughed, thinking that starting rounds at this outlandish hour must be a joke (it wasn't). The cardiothoracic surgical fellow, a grizzled PGY11, warned me that the attending surgeon would ask me my college major and if it were something related to science, tell me it was boring and ignore me for the rest of the case. I was a biochemistry major and so, as he poked at a child's heart the size of a walnut, I stood in silence for hours, uncomfortable, clueless, lightheaded, and bored.

I was tuning out, wishing I were anywhere else. Mostly, I was thinking about my couch, where I would curl up with a box of Honey Nut Cheerios and the latest episode of *ER* that evening, when I realized that he and the fellow were discussing the impact of the surgical plan on the baby's physical and emotional development. With a start, I realized that I had almost missed out on this opportunity. While I might have been ignored, I could still learn. The particular anatomy of the eponymous shunts they discussed eluded me then (and still does now). Still, I was humbled that they considered both the surgical complexity as well as the emotional development of the tiny human being on their operating table.

It was a fascinating glimpse into the world of pediatric cardiothoracic surgery; more than anatomy and sutures and endless dissection. This highly trained surgeon had sacrificed the greater part of his young adulthood to master the art of miniature heart manipulation. While he clearly didn't care about me, he really cared about this infant. This experience taught me that I could learn from anyone, even from someone who did not seem to like me. I resolved never to treat my students as children who should be seen and not heard. I also resolved to strive to learn from every attending physician I worked with because bad behavior can be as instructive as good and every interaction can be a lesson. Never tune out, always pay attention, and learn from both the good and bad encounters.

How do you get the most out of every medical school rotation? The secret to thriving in the ever-changing world of medical school rotations includes three tenets:

(1) Feign enthusiasm
(2) Commit to the rotation
(3) Accept that the price of service is scut.

1.2.1 Feign Enthusiasm

When I was a medical student, senior medical students and residents would advise me to show enthusiasm. I would grimace and assure them that everyone could see through the "gunners." Now, on the other side of the relationship, I cannot tell which students are genuine and which are faking it, so the argument of insincerity holds no water.

In addition, enthusiasm is a self-fulfilling prophecy. Like the chicken-egg conundrum, do you smile because you're happy or are you happy because you smile? If you pretend to be enthusiastic about the differential diagnosis of postpartum hemorrhage, postpartum hemorrhage will become more exciting to you. In addition, every resident, fellow, and attending physician who works with you on your clinical rotations is not paid to do so. In many ways, their lives would be easier if they didn't have to teach medical students: longer lunch breaks, shorter rounds, fewer teaching sessions. They do it because they're expected to and because they love it. Teaching a student who is excited to learn makes the teacher want to do more: enthusiasm begets better learning and better teaching.

Enthusiasm is contagious: by showing interest, you can transform a lackadaisical teacher into one willing to share their tips, tricks, and pearls for best patient care. I worked with a surgical resident who treated me like an appendix; she did not need me and were I removed, she would not have missed me. I tagged along with her on call nights as required and expressed genuine wonder at her ability to soothe distraught patients in the pre-operative area while juggling pages, consults, and admissions with equanimity. Her demeanor slowly transformed from long-suffering to tolerant and, finally, pleasant. She guided me through suture lacerations and showed me the best way to assess an acute abdomen. Though we were never buddies, I learned from her, initially from observation and later, luckily, through instruction.

Will showing your appreciation and sharing your enthusiasm always work? Of course not; nothing, not even rabies, is 100% effective in achieving its goal. Either way, however, it's a win–win situation: be kind and open and you will learn from what your residents and attending physicians do wrong or from what they do right.

Enthusiasm also begets concentration. Even the pretense of enthusiasm and paying attention takes effort. This effort at appearing to pay attention will focus your concentration so you actually will be paying attention. You will grasp more of the details and context, resulting in greater understanding and retention.

Finally, over time, enthusiasm will become second-nature. You will realize that there is always something to learn. You will naturally try to place new information and experiences in a clinically relevant context and improve your availability to care for patients. You will look forward to every rotation as an opportunity to become a better physician. Yes, you will encounter plenty of sticks in the mud—but you don't have to be one yourself.

1.2.2   Commit to the Rotation

It's hard to fathom in the thick of medical school, but medicine becomes so specialized that medical school may be the last time you deliver a baby, assist in the repair a ruptured abdominal aortic aneurysm, or evaluate a patient with a bowel perforation after colonoscopy. Pretend that, after medical school, you will be forced to go into whatever rotation you're currently on. You will pay far more attention than if you write off the rotations as something you'll never see or use again.

During my psychiatric rotation in medical school, I evaluated schizophrenic patients having a psychotic breaks, performed consultations on hospitalized patients with delirium, and rotated through the dementia unit of a long-term care facility. Decades later, when I evaluate patients with a change in mental status, I still use the knowledge I gained from that rotation. Based on that experience, I can distinguish psychosis, delirium, and dementia and formulate a management plan. Knowledge is never wasted, and everything counts as experience.

1.2.3   The Price of Service is Scut

For every bit of service, there is scut. On my neurosurgical rotation, back in the days of paper charts, the intern had me write skeleton notes for all his patients every morning. I would gather a sheaf of hospital notepaper, stamped with the names of the 20-odd patients on service, and write in the overnight vital signs, morning labs, and operative date, leaving space for the intern to add the subjective, exam, and plan. The administrative load was annoying, yet by easing his burden of paperwork, he had more free time. Lucky for me, he used this free time to teach: thanks to him, I learned the finer points of diagnosing appendicitis and cholecystitis during lulls on call nights.

Carrying the bag of bandage supplies on the vascular surgery rotation, holding retractors, removing sutures—all scut. Doing scut is the best way to make yourself less superfluous and more useful. By being a useful member of the team, you are more likely to be taught and more likely to learn. Scut can lead to more teaching and more experience.

A caveat: know what's scut, and what's not. Picking up dry cleaning, washing cars, watching toddlers—you will hopefully never experience these outlandish requests. Still, draw the line between scut that is medical (appropriate) and non-medical (not appropriate). If faced with scut that makes you feel more like a personal assistant, reach out to your program director for advice and assistance.

1.3   Final Thoughts

Medical school cannot, and should not, feel easy—but it should feel worthwhile. Identify a strategy/system that allows you to embrace the light at the end of the memorization tunnel. Celebrate the joys of finally appreciating the poetry of medicine. Accept the fear and uncertainty of the clinical years but recognize the enormous privilege you have to observe and experience the many facets of medicine, all aimed at making people feel better and saving lives.

References

Bemelmans L. Madeline. New York: Viking Press; 1963.
Fadiman A. The spirit catches you and you fall down: a Hmong child, her American doctors, and the collision of two cultures. Farrar, Straus, and Giroux; 1997.
Verghese A. My own country: a doctor's story (1st Vintage books). Vintage Books; 1995, 1994.

Chapter 2
Becoming Fluent in Medicine

When you finally get to speak on your medical school rotations, how do you shine? This chapter will cover formal oral and written presentations, step-by-step.

Instead of worrying, I compensated for my lack of quick thinking under stress with my secret weapon, a system of advanced preparation. If I were assigned a patient, I could and would know everything about that patient. By knowing everything and preparing my patient presentations coherently, I could shine. If you put in the time to prepare for rounds, you will learn to think clearly. If you think clearly, you will speak clearly. If you speak clearly, you will inspire trust and provide optimal patient care.

This chapter will cover formal oral and written presentations, step-by-step. I know what you're thinking: the kind of presentation expected on a rheumatology consult rotation is different from that expected in the medical intensive care unit or a general surgery service. Yes and no: a comprehensive, clearly organized, concise, and succinct presentation is always welcome. A vascular surgery attending once extended his hand to shake mine after I presented a patient as a third-year medical student. Was I a gifted future vascular surgeon? As the student who openly winced when faced with dry gangrene and felt lightheaded at the sight of an open abdomen—no. Yet I could present a patient, with advanced preparation, fluently and clearly, and any experienced physician (especially a surgeon) could appreciate this.

While you may tailor your approach for various specialties—skim over the family history for a patient on the trauma surgery service and focus more on this when rotating through oncology—always go back to the basics of same steps, in the same order, every time. The formal structure was created for a reason: it makes it easy to grasp the essentials of a complex patient. The structure will never let you down. Even when other team members are more casual, stay formal and stay focused. A formal presentation need not be longer than an informal, meandering, disorganized diatribe. Rather, sticking to your script helps you to be assured, eloquent, and knowledgeable. You may be inexperienced but you should never be unprepared.

M. Kittleson, *Mastering the Art of Patient Care*,
https://doi.org/10.1007/978-3-031-20920-8_2

2.1 Oral Presentations

2.1.1 The Identifying Statement

The goal is not to surprise your listeners (other medical students, residents, fellows, and attending physicians) with a mystery case. The goal is to offer a concise and cohesive review of the patient's presentation so listeners grasp the necessary information to diagnose and treat the patient. Thus, the identifying statement places the patient in context for the listener. It is succinct, complete, and relevant.

Model: This is a <age> <sex> with *<relevant* past medical history> who presents with a <duration> history of <symptom> admitted for <diagnosis>.

Bad: "This is a complex 57-year-old gentleman with hypertension, diabetes, prostate cancer, osteoarthritis, and peptic ulcer disease who presents with chest pain.
     Why bad?

– "Complex" doesn't tell the listener anything except that you were too lazy to distill the information for them.
– How is prostate cancer and osteoarthritis relevant to a presenting symptom of chest pain? Again, this signals to the listener that you didn't bother to helpfully organize the information. They will be distracted as they try to link the unrelated litany of medical problems and miss other parts of your presentation.
– The admitting diagnosis is missing. The presentation isn't a treasure hunt. Make it easy for the listener to learn everything about the patient in an efficient manner.

     Good: "This is a 57-year-old gentleman with a history of diabetes and hypertension who presents with a 3-day history of exertional chest discomfort no longer relieved by rest admitted for unstable angina."
     Why good?

– The listener is given a precise snapshot of relevant details including medical problems and symptoms which support the admitting diagnosis.

2.1.2 The History of Present Illness

There is no better place to highlight your talents as a competent diagnostician than the History of Present Illness (HPI). You will weave facts into a clear history that supports your diagnosis. The patient's chronology is not necessarily a medically relevant chronology. You must synthesize, not regurgitate, information. The patient may tell you their story in a random order. You will sift through the information to create a history that makes medical sense. You may slot some facts into the history of present illness, some into the past medical history, some into social history, some into review of systems. Patients report facts—you organize ideas.

Model:

(1) **Set the stage: describe relevant PMH**
(2) **Start at the beginning: establish a baseline with the usual state of health**
(3) **Describe nature, duration, frequency, precipitating/exacerbating/relieving factors, associated symptoms, pertinent positives, and pertinent negatives**
(4) **End at the end: where did the patient present (clinic, ED via paramedics, ambulance, transfer from another hospital) and why did they choose that mode of presentation?**

Example: Mr. X was diagnosed with a nonischemic cardiomyopathy in 2005 when he presented with decompensated heart failure and echocardiogram showed ejection 25%. Coronary angiogram showed no coronary artery disease. Given a history of heart failure in his father and brother, he was presumed to have a familial cardiomyopathy [*Relevant PMH*]. He was managed by his primary cardiologist and did well for years. He was in this usual state of health, able to walk 3 miles without shortness of breath, until 2 weeks prior to presentation [*Establish a baseline*]. At that time, he noted shortness of breath on inclines. For the past week, he has not exercised due to shortness of breath and leg swelling. For the past two nights, he has had shortness of breath while lying flat. He reports that he has missed doses of diuretics occasionally for the past 2 weeks because he was concerned about the impact of frequent urination on his busy work and travel schedule [*Symptoms with pertinent positives*]. He saw his cardiologist for an urgent appointment. His cardiologist referred him to the emergency department [*Mode of presentation*].

Why is this HPI good? By clearly and concisely offering all relevant details, you can determine if the appropriate evaluation was performed at the time of diagnosis. You have a sense of how sick he is based on the trajectory of his symptoms and mode of presentation. You have insight into the cause of his decompensation which can direct care and future preventive measures. Apply this model to any patient and you will provide team members with the best opportunity to provide optimal patient care.

2.1.3 The Past Medical History

The PMH is not a laundry list of random medical conditions. The PMH is curated, organized, and stratified to make sense. When you start out, you won't know what facts are necessary to stratify the severity of each PMH item. With experience, you will get a better sense of this. A way to short-cut this experience: review notes from the relevant consultants in the chart. The pulmonologist, endocrinologist, infectious disease specialist, and cardiologist will likely include the relevant facts that guide management in their notes—learn from them through their notes!

Also, every item in the PMH is fair game for your attending to assess your fund of knowledge on rounds. Make sure you understand what you're saying—look things up—know the facts!

Model:

(1) **When diagnosed**
(2) **The most recent parameters that describe severity**
(3) **How it's been treated**
(4) **Who follows the patient (if there is a particular specialist involved).**

Bad: PMH: COPD, diabetes, HIV, atrial fibrillation.
Good:
COPD: diagnosed in ___, PFTs in ___ showed ___, prior hospitalizations/intubations/steroid pulses ___; followed by Dr. ___ [if pulmonologist involved].
Diabetes: diagnosed in ___, evidence of nephropathy/neuropathy/retinopathy___, last Hgb A1c ___ in ___, followed by Dr. ___ [if endocrinologist involved}.
HIV diagnosed in ___, prior opportunistic infections include ___, most recent viral load ___ in ___, most recent CD4 count ___ in ___, followed by Dr. ___ [if infectious disease specialist involved].
Atrial fibrillation: diagnosed in ___, (a)symptomatic, paroxysmal/persistent/permanent, managed with rate control/rhythm control, prior cardioversions/ablations in ___, CHA2DS2-VASc score ___, on/not on anticoagulation (if not as indicated, then why), followed by Dr. ___ [if cardiologist/electrophysiologist involved].

Why is this PMH good? The reader will now have a great understanding of the patient's medical conditions. A bonus: you will have learned about the management of COPD, diabetes, HIV, and atrial fibrillation by putting together the important parameters of severity for each condition.

2.1.4   Medications

This is straightforward, right? How can you go wrong with a list of medications? You can, if you present only trade names, neglect to report dose/frequency/duration, and don't know the indication of every medication on the list. Let's go over why these details are important.

There are many advantages to presenting generic names over trade names. First, the generic names for medications have the same suffix so you will become familiar with drug classes by knowing them; -pril for ACE inhibitors, -olol for beta-blockers, and so on. Second, since generic medications are almost always just as effective and less expensive, choose them first. The only reason to use a trade medication when the generic one is as effective is because you have been swayed by the marketing strategies of the pharmaceutical companies—or because you cannot remember the generic alternatives since you always refer to medications by trade names.

That's not to say there aren't instances where you will rely on brand-name medications. If you have free samples in clinic, you may offer your patient a month's supply of the free brand-name version as you work to make the medication more affordable based on their prescription plan or patient assistance programs. In addition, you will need to know both names as the patient may be more familiar with the trade name. Neither of these corollaries, however, should prevent you from reporting the generic names in your formal presentation.

Report the dose and frequency of every medication. The dose and frequency can offer insight into the stability and severity of the condition being treated. A patient with heart failure who tolerates carvedilol 25 mg twice daily is more stable than one who can take only 3.125 mg twice daily. A patient with neuropathy who takes gabapentin 600 mg three times a day has more severe symptoms than one whose neuropathy is controlled with 100 mg at bedtime. Knowledge of the dose and frequency of medication administration will allow to you better formulate a management plan.

Report the duration of antibiotics. Is the patient being treated for an uncomplicated urinary tract infection or a cardiovascular implantable electronic device infection? Reporting the duration of antibiotic therapy communicates helpful information for those caring for the patient and helps you learn the protocols for various infections.

Know the indication for every medication on the patient's list. If you don't know, look it up! If you follow this rule for every patient, you will shine as a trainee. You will show initiative and demonstrate an effective technique for self-education. Far more importantly, if you maintain this practice, you will strengthen the habit of directed learning that will serve you, and your patients, throughout your career. Good habits start in medical school: you can start with your oral and written patient presentations.

2.1.5 *Allergies*

This is another straightforward item though there are still pitfalls. Don't just list allergies. Specify the specific interaction, as many intolerances end up on the allergy list. Angioedema from an ACE inhibitor versus cough from an ACE inhibitor are not the same. You may attempt an ACE inhibitor again in the latter patient but never in the former. Intolerances and allergies warrant different management strategies.

Model: Drug name and details of allergy/intolerance/side effects and notes for future use.

Bad: Allergies: ACE inhibitors, prednisone, amoxicillin.
Good: Allergies: ACE inhibitors → cough (intolerable, resolved after cessation).
Prednisone → weight gain (patient-reported side effect; OK to use).
Amoxicillin → diarrhea (patient-reported side effect; OK to use).

Why is this allergy list good? Sometimes patients with heart failure have a cough due to congestion, not the ACE inhibitor-related increase in bradykinin resulting in bronchospasm. Documenting that the cough was intolerable and resolved after the medication was stopped helps other clinicians know whether to re-attempt the medication and how serious the reaction was.

Prednisone causes weight gain; that's a side effect, not an allergy or intolerance. If the patient is someday diagnosed with giant cell arteritis, there should not be an alert in the chart about prednisone. Corticosteroids would be indicated to treat giant cell arteritis and no serious adverse effects would ensue.

Having amoxicillin on the allergy list without additional information is dangerous; is there a history of anaphylaxis and all penicillins should be avoided? In this case, no: maybe the patient subsequently undergoes a valve replacement and now needs amoxicillin prophylaxis for dental procedures. This would be perfectly fine; the potential for diarrhea would be unlikely given the single-dose prophylaxis recommended for dental procedures.

2.1.6 Social History

Take the time to take a social history—though, really, it takes almost no time at all and the return on investment (satisfaction for you and your patient) is great. When I was a cardiology fellow on the consult service, my attending would ask, without fail, where every patient was born and raised. When I told him, he would take an atlas off his bookshelf and locate the patient's hometown. Then, when we rounded on the patient, he would ask a few questions about where they were from. With this simple habit, I learned a lot about the geography of the Mid-Atlantic states, and he showed how much he cared about and thereby strengthened the patient physician bond.

Glean a nonmedical fact from every patient because it is these nonmedical facts that transform every patient into a human being. These details transform the cold and sterile scientific world of the hospital into a warmer place where people are more than a collection of their diseases.

Model: S/he was born and raised in _____. S/he works at _____. S/he lives with _____. (Bonus points for pets/names). S/he has _____ children and ____ grandchildren. (Bonus points for names/ages). Cigarette use _____. Alcohol use _____. Drug use _____.

Bad: no smoking/drugs/alcohol.

Good: She was born and raised in Illinois and moved to California at the age of 10. She works in human resources for a law firm and lives at home with her wife of 14 years. They have two children, aged 10 and 12. She smoked cigarettes, 1 ppd for 10 years, and quit 11 years ago. She drinks 1–2 beers on Friday and Saturday nights. She does not use illicit drugs.

Why is this social history good? The bad minimalist approach above robs you of your opportunity to know the patient. A more complete version provides an important sense of who she is as well as her habits that may impact her health. In addition, when you read your note later, trying to place one patient among thousands, you will have context to guide you.

When it comes to alcohol, I ask, "Do you drink alcohol?" Open-ended questions are important, but if the answer is yes, I will then ask, "A few drinks a day or a few drinks a week?" By presuming that the default is more, you will allow the patient to offer a more truthful estimate of their alcohol intake without judgment.

Knowing the right way to take a sexual history is important too. I saw an internist instead of a pediatrician for the first time for a routine physical examination before heading off to college. He asked, "Do you have a boyfriend?" and when I said no, he moved on to my family history. Now, I had no sexual history to speak of at the time, but what if I had? That single question, rife with expectation, closed the door to any further responses.

When taking a sexual history, keep the questions open-ended and non-judgmental. Start the conversation with, "Are you comfortable talking about your sexual history? I understand these questions are personal, but they are important for your health." If the patient is open to discussion, focus open-ended questions on the 5 P's: partners, practices, protection from sexually-transmitted illnesses, past history of sexually-transmitted illnesses, and pregnancy intention. Let the patient's responses guide you.

2.1.7 Family History

When you take a family history, the reported cause of death might not be the medical cause of death, as in "dad died of a heart attack" could mean anything from ventricular fibrillation arrest to myocardial infarction to pulmonary embolism to stroke or subarachnoid hemorrhage. When you record illnesses and causes of death of parents, siblings, or children, be sure to specify if these are reported causes of death or confirmed by post-mortem examination. Because genetic conditions have variable penetrance and expressivity, it may take a 3-generation family history for a pattern to emerge. If you sense a pattern emerging, take the time to ask about cousins, aunts, uncles, and grandparents too.

Model: who (bare minimum: parents/siblings), how old when diagnosed/died, cause of death, how diagnosed/confirmed (when applicable)

Consider this example below:

Bad: cousin died of a heart attack at 34.

Why is this family history bad? It's bad because it's incomplete. Did the patient's cousin have a myocardial infarction, or something else? Did he have a history of heart disease or cardiac testing or intervention? How was the diagnosis confirmed?

Good: brother died at 23 in a drowning accident, paternal cousin died at 34 of a reported "heart attack" (found dead at home, no post-mortem examination performed), paternal uncle died at 45 in a car accident (as the driver, no other cars involved).

Why is this family history good? Because more probing questions about the cousin's death were asked, a diagnosis of sudden cardiac death was made. The recognition of sudden cardiac death in the cousin then triggered additional questions. Sudden death may manifest as drowning or car accidents. Asking directed questions about potential modes of sudden cardiac death revealed a disturbing and unexpected pattern—one that could have significant implications for the patient's evaluation and management.

This example is based on my experience with a patient referred to me with a murmur and left ventricular hypertrophy on echocardiogram. From reading the prior notes, I thought there may a history of premature coronary artery disease based on the description of the cousin's death. By asking the right questions, a more accurate picture emerged. This was crucial as a family history like this in a patient with hypertrophic cardiomyopathy tips the scales towards implantation of a defibrillator for primary prevention of sudden cardiac death.

The family history is important for more than identifying heritable conditions. The family history also allows you to gain insight into the patient's fears and concerns. A patient came to see me because he was worried about his heart. He was 45 years old with no medical problems and exercised regularly without symptoms. Nonetheless, he was scared that he would not survive to see his infant daughter start kindergarten.

What might have seemed like anxiety out of proportion to his medical condition made far more sense after I elicited a particularly grim family history: his father and four uncles had all died from coronary artery disease before the age of 50. Armed with this insight, we discussed the environmental versus genetic impact of different forms of heart disease and made a concrete action plan to identify and mitigate his risk factors. Without this family history, I would not have been able to provide optimal patient care.

2.1.8 Review of Systems

The ROS does not have to be long. Pertinent positives and pertinent negatives are in the HPI. Non-pertinent positives are in the ROS.

Model: non-pertinent positive symptoms

You might ask about a ton of items, but you need not report a ton of times—just the non-pertinent positives go here.

2.1.9 Physical Examination and Laboratories

The most important key to the presentation of the physical examination is: describe, don't editorialize. There will be plenty of opportunity to editorialize in the plan. In the objective portion of the presentation, provide only the facts. Here, your particular rotation plays a big role: the vascular surgeon will not want a detailed cognitive assessment and the oncologist will not care about every joint's range of motion. As you move from rotation to rotation, you will hone your skills at various parts of the physical examination that are crucial for that specialty. Still, no matter what, present in this order for best impact:

Model:

(1) **Organ systems in order: General appearance, Head/Eyes/Ears/Nose/Throat, Chest, Abdomen, Back, Rectal/Genitourinary, Extremities, Skin, Neurologic, Psychiatric**
(2) **Findings within the organ system in order: inspection, palpation, percussion, auscultation**
(3) **Level of detail appropriate for the patient's symptoms and the specialty.**

Bad: "The patient appears fatigued. I don't think he slept well. I will write him for a sleeping pill tonight. Oh, and the JVP 10 cm H_2O. He was 2L negative on Lasix. Lungs have decreased breath sounds at the bases. The CXR didn't show an effusion, though. I can check an ultrasound to assess for an effusion? Yes, and abdomen is soft. Pulses are within normal limits. The neuro examination is nonfocal."

Why is this description of the physical examination bad? First, too much stream of consciousness. The listener will get distracted and once you lose your listener's interest, it's hard to regain it. Second, "within normal limits" and "nonfocal" are just disingenuous ways of saying "I actually didn't examine this body part." Instead of "within normal limits," describe what's normal. Instead of "nonfocal," leave it out.

Good: "The patient is in no apparent distress. JVP 10 cm H_2O. Lungs have decreased breath sounds at the bases. Heart is regular with no murmurs or gallops. Abdomen is soft without organomegaly or tenderness. Extremities are warm without edema".

Why is this description of the physical examination good? It is organized and relevant with appropriate positives and negatives to give the listener an accurate assessment of the degree of decompensated heart failure.

2.1.10 Assessment

The assessment is the summary statement. It resembles the initial identifying statement with more detail because your listener is now primed for more relevant details.

Model: This is a \<age\> \<sex\> with *\<relevant* past medical history\> who presents with a \<duration\> history of \<symptom\>. He was noted to have \<relevant physical exam findings\> and \<relevant lab/study findings\>. He was admitted for \<diagnosis\>.

Example: "This is a 57-year-old gentleman with a history of diabetes and hypertension who presents with a 3-day history of exertional chest discomfort no longer relieved by rest. On examination, he was chest-pain free with JVP 4 cm, no murmurs or gallops, and no edema. Troponin was 0.04 ng/ml and EKG showed new inferolateral ST depressions. He was admitted for unstable angina."

This is an outstanding assessment because it lets the listener know how you made the diagnosis and how sick the patient is. You have culled together the important details into a clear summary. An experienced physician can make a complicated patient appear simple; an inexperienced physician can make a simple patient appear complicated. You can model an experienced physician if you have a system. Thorough preparation and organized templates will bring clarity to your thinking and your presentations.

2.1.11 Plan

When I was a sub-intern in the medical intensive care unit, I would spend 45 min pre-rounding on a single patient. I gathered vital signs and laboratory values, read consult notes and imaging reports, and spent the bulk of my time writing out my plan organized by system. This way, I wouldn't forget anything or fumble on rounds. As an intern, I would spend 10–15 min per patient gathering data and working out my plan. As a resident, I allowed myself 5 min per patient. As an attending, I need 1–2 min. (More in Chap. 7 on why pre-rounding doesn't end when internship does.) Putting the time in early in your training will give you experience and pays dividends later in your career.

Model:

(1) **State the system**
(2) **State the problem within that system**
(3) **Offer an assessment of whether the problem is getting better, worse, or staying the same**
(4) **Provide the plan for the day, focusing on the rationale, the goal of the day, the goal of the hospitalization, and the tools to achieve that goal.**

Bad: "Cardiac—Heart failure. The patient is on Lasix 80 IV BID. Continue to monitor".

Why bad? There is no assessment of the severity of trajectory of the HF course. There is no plan, just a statement of what the current therapy is. "Continue to monitor" is not a plan. "Continue to monitor" is a cop-out. If you never allow yourself to utter (or write) the phrase "continue to monitor," your plans will automatically exponentially improve. Have an opinion on patient management. The patients trusts you to make a plan for them. Formulating an incorrect plan (with a rationale you can use to support it) is preferable to having no plan at all. Having an opinion on how to manage a problem means that you are actively attempting to synthesize medical knowledge into clinical judgment.

Someday, you will be confident in your judgement. Until then, you will practice honing your judgment by reasoning through clinical scenarios and making decisions. When you take ownership and make decisions, you will gain valuable experience. Attendings are there to help you—avail yourself of this safety net!

Bad: "Cardiac—Heart failure. Do you want to continue Lasix 80 mg IV BID?".

Why bad? Be a Captain, not a Waiter (more on this in Chap. 8). It is not your job to solicit opinions; it is your job to have opinions (more on Captains and Waiters in Chap. 8). By soliciting an opinion from your attending physician rather than having one, you are abdicating the ownership that is the key to gaining judgment and experience. Take the leap of courage and have a plan while you still have the safety net of your attending physician to guide you. An easy way to take ownership in baby steps: before you ask your attending physician their opinion, offer your own: "I think we should continue Lasix 80 mg IV BID to maintain the current level of diuresis. Do you agree?".

Bad: "Cardiac—Heart failure. I believe the patient is on Lasix 80 mg IV BID."

Why bad? Is a Lasix dose something that requires faith? Do you believe the Lasix is at a given dose, or do you know it? There is never an excuse for hedging. It's far better to say, "I'm sorry. I don't remember the Lasix dose but I'll look it up now." Precision is better than imprecision and honesty is preferable to hedging to appear precise. The latter fools no one, and you cheat yourself out of a proper learning experience and the patient out of a physician who learns to be precise and organized.

Good: "Cardiac—Heart failure. Volume. Patient remains volume overloaded with JVP 12 cm H$_2$O and 2+ edema [*the problem*]. He was only 1 L negative despite Lasix 40 IV BID [*assessment of the problem*]. The goal for the day is to make him 2–3 L negative [*goal for the day*] and I anticipate he is still 8L above his dry weight [*goal for hospitalization*]. We will increase Lasix to 80 IV BID [*tool to achieve the goal*]."

Why good? The problem is succinctly outlined, assessed, and plan made. The plan uses tools (Lasix) and goals (I/O). Even if you're wrong—the JVP is not elevated, the edema is from something else, and more diuresis is not needed—you will still benefit from the exercise in medical reasoning. You will have a better understanding of why your reasoning was wrong and will be less likely to make the same mistake again. Presenting an organized and precise plan is a skill that is easy to master if you follow a system: use the template incorporating assessment, tools, and goals. Adherence to this model will provide you with valuable experience in clinical judgment and medical decision-making.

There are certain components that should be a part of every plan, no matter if the patient is admitted with cardiogenic shock to the intensive care unit or diverticulitis to the medicine ward. These are:

(1) Tubes, lines, and drains: Does the patient have any, and do they need them? Coco Chanel said, "Before you leave the house, look in the mirror and take one thing off." When caring for a patient, channel your inner Coco Chanel. Before you leave the room, look at the patient and determine if something can come off, whether it be a Foley catheter, nasal cannula, or a central line. The fewer indwelling catheters, the less chance for infections and complications. As important, the fewer unnecessary indwelling catheters, the more the patient feels like a healthy person who is progressing towards discharge. Help your patients feel as healthy as possible.

(2) Family: Is the patient and their family appropriately updated on the patient's course? Is there a need for a family meeting to discuss prognosis and goals of

care? This is most relevant for patients who are critically ill. Family updates are also crucial for patients with delirium or dementia where caregivers are an essential part of the treatment team.

(3) Criteria for transfer out of the intensive care unit or discharge from the hospital. The hospital discharge is a plant that you must water for it to bloom. Enumerate daily what the patient needs to accomplish to achieve the ultimate goal of leaving the hospital. This will help you to focus on the big picture amidst all the minor details and it highlights the patient's trajectory: are they moving towards, or farther away, from this ultimate goal?

2.1.12 The Daily Presentation

The daily presentation will be a curtailed version of your formal oral presentation. You'll start with a one-liner that encapsulates all that is relevant about the patient's relevant past history, presenting symptoms, admitting diagnosis, and hospital course.

Before delving into the classic SOAP format (Subjective, Objective, Assessment, and Plan), present the overnight events. Overnight events should tell a story: beginning, middle, and end.

Model:

(1) **The event**
(2) **The symptoms**
(3) **The tests performed (and results if available)**
(4) **The treatments provided**
(5) **The patient's response**

Wrong: Overnight events: the patient had a fever.

Right: Overnight events: The patient had a temperature of 102.4 F associated with a new cough. A chest X-ray showed a new left lower lobe infiltrate. A sputum gram stain and culture were stent and he was started empirically on ceftriaxone. He subsequently defervesced with temperature 98.9 F and is feeling better this morning.

More pointers on mastering the oral presentation.

2.1.13 Keep to Your Script

The key to clarity is keeping to your script. The script is your system for success. The more organized you are, the more eloquent you will be. Presentations are not the time for extemporaneous soliloquies. (And let's be honest, there is never a good time for those. You will not trick your attending physician into thinking you are smarter or more prepared just because you take longer to present your patient.) Remember, the sign of an experienced physician is that they can make a complex patient appear simple. How do they do this? They employ a system with a template. Same order, same phraseology, every time. Having a system and a concrete action plan will allow you to practice medicine calmly.

Your audience (the residents, fellows, attendings—your evaluators) listen to presentation after presentation. They are conditioned to process facts in order. If you present out of order, your audience will be confused, distracted, miss information as they try to piece together disparate facts, and soon lose faith in you. If you use this system to present in a clear order, your audience will absorb more. You will be polished and prepared. Patients benefit, you benefit: win–win.

2.1.14 Know Your Patient

There is never an excuse for not knowing the relevant facts. Anything in the patient's PMH or medication list that you present is fair game. If you say the patient has post-transplant lymphoproliferative disorder, you'd better have looked it up and know how that diagnosis is relevant to your patient's presentation. If you say the patient is receiving rituximab, you should know what this is and why they're on it. Knowing the relevant facts serves many purposes: you demonstrate initiative and you're also learning in context, which is the best way to learn and grow your experience.

Consider yourself lucky: not all of us trained in the era of the internet search engines. I remember suddenly realizing, on rounds while a fellow medical student was presenting their patient, that I had failed to look up the mechanism of the interaction between azathioprine and allopurinol. I knew my attending physician would ask about it and that I could never race to the medical library and back in time to look it up in *Harrisons Principles of Internal Medicine*. I had to frantically search my memory banks in vain and resigned to come up short when my attending questioned me on rounds. You, on the other hand, can calmly search UpToDate or your favorite resource on your phone; you can be prepared and confident by the time you present your patient. Take advantage of the wealth of knowledge at your fingertips to provide the optimal patient care.

2.1.15 Practice Makes Perfect

Practice, practice, practice. How do you get to Carnegie Hall? How do you ace your rotation? You get the picture. Write it all out and practice to yourself, your cat, your roommate, your mom on FaceTime. Practice never made anyone imperfect: the more you practice, the closer you will be to becoming a competent physician.

2.2   The Art of the Note

As you master the art of the oral presentation, you will also be mastering the art of the written note. There are many reasons to write an accurate, clear, comprehensive, and consistent note: (1) you must think clearly to write clearly so writing a clear note will reinforce your clear thinking; (2) if your notes are reliable and well-written, team communication and thus patient care is optimized; and (3) as an intern and beyond, you are judged, forevermore, by the quality of your notes, so grasp every opportunity to shine!

The art of the note follows many of the same rules of the oral presentation outlined above. Here are the pitfalls to avoid so that you can ensure your notes always reliably and accurately communicate best practices to promote optimal patient care.

2.2.1   Make It Make Sense

Inconsistency is the bane of note-readers' existence. With the dawn of electronic medical records, the frustration of illegible handwritten notes has been replaced with the unintelligible copy-forwarded notes that are annoying at best and dangerous at worst. Consider a note that says the patient has no symptoms in the subjective section, describes him as intubated/sedated in the physical exam section, and reports that he will be discharged home in the next few days in the plan section. The reader immediately assumes that the note is rife with other serious inconsistencies. The reader then assumes that the note, and its writer, are not to be trusted. Inconsistencies put patients' lives in danger.

How to combat against this? Read your note through, in its entirety. Of course, you may be overwhelmed by the thought of doing this if you write 15 copy-forwarded notes daily. In that case, just pick one note on one patient per day and read their note through start to finish. I suspect you will be so aghast by the embarrassing inconsistencies that you will be inspired to read through the rest of your notes in rapid succession. There is more than pride at stake. Inaccurate notes impair communication among health care professionals, and miscommunication puts patients' lives at risk.

You will also scroll through interminable and often meaningless tables of problem lists compiled piecemeal by everyone who touches the electronic medical record. Which leads me to the next tip.

2.2.2   Brevity is the Soul of a Good Note

What's the best way to write a concise yet comprehensive note? On an admission note, except for the smart phrases for medications and vital signs, type out the rest yourself: the HPI, PMH, social history, family history, ROS, exam, assessment, and plan. On a follow-up note for a patient you're picking up at the start of a new rotation, do the same thing, focusing on crafting a succinct one-liner assessment and short paragraph summary of the hospital course (that you will update daily to ensure it remains succinct and accurate). This exercise, of eschewing the dreaded piles of smart phrases and copy-forwards from other people's work, will mean that (1) the information is accurate because you had to type it in yourself; and (2) it will be considerably shorter, also because you had to type it in yourself.

Is this a lot to ask? Yes, it is. Does it take a lot of work? Yes, at first. Do I practice what I preach? Of course! When I'm on call for the weekend, I spend Saturday rewriting notes so I'm convinced they're accurate. Sunday goes more quickly as my accurate template is established, and I can be secure in the knowledge that troubling inconsistencies will not place patients' lives in danger.

You will discover that the effort to write accurate, clear, consistent, and comprehensive notes is worth it. Ensuring your notes are readable, succinct, accurate, and consistent will serve you well for decades to come. You will earn a reputation of a thorough and conscientious physician whom others trust to care for their patients. Most importantly, your patients will receive optimal care.

2.2.3 If You Write It, You Own It

Just as anything in your oral presentation is fair game for questions, don't write anything in your note that doesn't make sense to you. If you record that the patient is receiving tocilizumab for rheumatoid arthritis, you must look up the mechanism of action and indication and even add this information to your note for future reference. By ensuring you know what everything means, you will learn more and your note will be a useful reference for your readers.

2.2.4 Close the Loop

Imagine you perform a consult, and your plan indicates that your final recommendations depend on pending test results. What happens when those test results return? Do you write an addendum to your note, or a new note, indicating your final recommendations? Yes, you do. Because if you don't, then the person reviewing the chart (days, weeks, or months later) has no way to piece together the story of the patient because critical details, like your final expert assessment, are missing.

When I perform a preoperative cardiac evaluation, sometimes I recommend additional testing. Decades ago, I saw a patient once who required surgery for laryngeal cancer but reported new dyspnea on exertion with a loud murmur on examination. I was concerned that he might have symptomatic severe aortic stenosis with potential implications for the timing of surgery. The echocardiogram, done a few days later, fortunately showed only moderate aortic stenosis and I told the relieved patient he was fine to proceed with surgery as planned. However, in my inexperience, I did not document this in my note and over the next week as the date of surgery approached, received 4 urgent calls from the surgeon's office, the surgeon, the anesthesiologist, and the primary care physician to confirm the patient's fitness to proceed. I remedied my error with an addendum to my consult note, but my lack of documentation could have delayed an important surgery. Now, I know better: I close the loop with documentation of my final assessment and recommendations.

Leave nothing hanging. By the time someone has reviewed your notes, there should be no lingering questions regarding the evaluation and management plan. Mysteries are for mystery writers; your note should never be a puzzle that needs to be solved by another member of the healthcare team.

2.2.5   Useful Tips and Tricks

To some, the note may be a medicolegal document. To others, the note serves a documentation for billing. To everyone, it is first and foremost a reference to communicate the information necessary to treat patients. If it fulfills this role, patients will receive the best of care and the medicolegal and billing requirements will naturally follow.

Report dates, not days. In the current era of copy-forward electronic notes, there is no better way to gain the distrust of your reader than to have phrases in your note like, "The patient was extubated yesterday" when the patient was in fact extubated two weeks prior. Words like yesterday, today, and tomorrow are meaningless in the age of electronic medical records. Instead, use dates. "The patient was extubated on 2/24/20."

Put important information in helpful places. Sure, the statin will be on the medication list—but would it be helpful to put it somewhere else too? The current ACC/AHA cholesterol guidelines recommend that patients with coronary artery disease achieve a 50% reduction in LDL on statin therapy. So, record the baseline fasting lipid panel off statin therapy, if available, and then record the most recent lipid panel with the name/dose of statin next to it. This allows the reader, and you, to assess the impact of the statin easily without having to search through multiple parts in the chart to synthesize the information.

If the patient is not on a medication that is the standard of care, document why. All patients with heart failure and reduced ejection fraction should be on sacubitril/valsartan. If your patient is not, document why: patient declined, angioedema, intolerance due to XYZ, etc. Provide the reader with all the answers to anticipated questions so they can seamlessly care for the patient.

2.2.6 Cringe-Worthy Phrases

There are certain phrases that, when present in the chart, immediately render the note suspect. These are cop-outs, nonspecific or inconsistent, which should be avoided at all costs.

To name just a few:

"Continue to monitor" as noted above, is not a concrete action plan. What are you monitoring? What parameters are you looking for and how will they change your management? If an issue is so stable that you can think of nothing to say except "continue to monitor" (such as daily assessment of creatinine in a patient with normal renal function) then omit this item from the plan.

If you need to monitor a parameter, then elaborate instead with an "if, then" statement. Don't write "Elevated creatinine: continue to monitor." Instead, write, "Elevated creatinine consistent with cardiorenal syndrome; plan is ongoing diuresis. If creatinine continues to rise, then we will place pulmonary artery catheter to document volume status and cardiac index and assess need for inotropic support."

"Follow up as outpatient" is not a plan. If a patient has a new renal mass found incidentally on a CT scan performed to evaluate diverticulitis, the plan is not "follow up as outpatient." The plan is "discussed with urology who feels there is no urgency to perform further imaging tests as an inpatient. The patient's internist is aware and a contrast CT has been ordered and coordinated with an outpatient urology appointment."

"Avoid nephrotoxins." So obvious as to be ridiculous; is anyone going to actively administer nephrotoxins to their patients? It is the job of the physician to determine which medications the patient might be on are nephrotoxins and avoid them. Better: "The patient takes ibuprofen as needed and used 3 doses yesterday. As NSAIDs are nephrotoxic and his renal function is worsening, ibuprofen should be discontinued."

"Gentle diuresis" This phrase is a sign that the physician is unsure of the patient's volume status and wishes to hedge their bets. Have an opinion: the patient is either wet, dry, or euvolemic. If wet, specify goal I/O for diuresis. If dry, specify goal I/O for fluid resuscitation. If euvolemic, specify diuretic dosage planned to achieve even fluid balance. If unsure, specify how you will become sure (perhaps a by placing a pulmonary artery catheter to assess filling pressures).

2.3 Final Thoughts

When I was a fellow, I sat down an intern who was rounding with me in the CCU. I gave him my spiel on the art of the oral presentation and the note just as one of my mentors from medical school had done for me. The intern was hesitant, fumbling, and uncertain, yet he was anxious to learn. He took copious notes and his presentations and clinical judgment improved steadily over the course of our month together. I offered him complimentary feedback and went on to my next rotation.

A few years later, he emailed me to let me know that he had been chosen as chief resident and been accepted at his first-choice cardiology fellowship program. He thanked me for mentoring him; he had employed my foolproof system of presentations to great fanfare and accolades from other team members. More importantly, having a system replaced the stress of uncertainty with the confidence of preparation and helped him experience the joy of medicine. My pointers in the CCU early in his internship provided him with a system. He was convinced that he otherwise would never have been chosen to be chief resident or matched in the cardiology program of his dreams.

I was happy to take some credit; after all, I planted the seed. He provided the fertile soil of motivation and the constant tending of diligence. You, too, are planting the seed of good habits in medicine and tending them with motivation and diligence. You are building the successful foundation of experience to provide optimal patient care.

Chapter 3
Your Career Path

Medical students are like pluripotent stem cells: master cells with infinite powers of differentiation. Pluripotent stem cells can turn into any cell or tissue in the body, from intestinal endothelium to neuroglia to cardiac myocytes. Just like that, a medical student may be transformed into a gastroenterologist, neurosurgeon, or cardiologist. Of course, the analogy ends there: pluripotent stem cells have endless capacity for self-renewal while medical students are, unfortunately, not immortal.

For a stem cell, differentiation occurs through the magic of cell–cell interactions and exposure to growth factors or cytokines. For a medical student, specialization happens as soon as a residency program is chosen. In medical school, my study partner and I essentially functioned as a shared brain. We studied together nightly for the medical licensing examination and had exactly the same fund of knowledge (though his ability to recite the coagulation cascade from memory always outstripped mine). He became a dermatologist, which didn't surprise me. He loved sorting skin findings by morphology, size, dermarcation, and distribution. His eyes lit up when we shadowed a dermatologist who explained the principle of Mohs micrographic surgery. We started out as a shared brain but now, after decades of specialization, our funds of knowledge barely overlap.

Pluripotent stem cells differentiate and medical students specialize, inspired not by cytokines and growth factors but by clinical rotations and mentors. The specialization process offers many decision points, all with the potential to bring you joy in medicine. Here is my advice for the various paths your career may take.

3.1 Research

Some medical students have a passion for direct patient care. Others are drawn to research, the chance to engage in investigation that may benefit patients on a larger scale. The best way to determine if research is the right path for you is to engage in research projects. In fact, even if you already think research is not the right path

M. Kittleson, *Mastering the Art of Patient Care*,
https://doi.org/10.1007/978-3-031-20920-8_3

for you, you should engage in research projects for perspective and experience. Two pieces of advice on how to pick the project: (1) pick the mentor, not the project; (2) start with research more basic in training than you plan to do in your career.

3.1.1 Pick the Mentor not the Project

As a college student, I had to decide between working in one of two labs for the summer. The first option was working with a principal investigator (PI) with a renowned track record of mentoring college students to greatness, though I was unfamiliar with his research focus and his lab was in a dingy building where I wouldn't have my own desk. The second option was working with a PI who was known to be distant and leave medical student mentoring to his post-doctoral students, though his research focus interested me, and his lab was in a brand-new facility where I would have my own desk for the summer.

It seems obvious in retrospect that I should have picked the first option, though I didn't; the idea of working on a cutting-edge research project in a shiny new facility appealed to me. Inexperienced though I was, I should have realized that, as a medical student, I would never be given a cutting-edge project. I had a great post-doc to guide me, though his mentorship mostly involved how to manage the mercurial temperament of the PI.

If I had worked for the other PI, would I have ended up loving basic science research? I doubt it. Still, I might have had a better experience learning about the analysis and implications of basic research on clinical science. The lesson: as a fledgling student of research, pay attention to the scuttlebutt of the trainee grapevine—potential PIs have reputations and track records for a reason—and focus on the mentor, not the research topic. For most trainees interested in gaining experience, it's not the project that matters, it's the mentor. The best opportunities will arise from a supportive mentor.

3.1.2 Start More Basic

The second important piece of advice: do research during your training that is one step more basic than you plan to do in your career. If you envision a career in clinical research, spend your dedicated research time as a fellow doing translational work. Why? First, translational research is ultimately the foundation of clinical research, so direct participation will give you a greater appreciation of where the ideas for clinical trials begin.

Second, it is nearly impossible to go "backwards" in research after your training is complete; you can't do clinical research as a fellow and expect to run a basic science laboratory as a faculty physician. Gain experience in something more basic than you anticipate you'll like. You may surprise yourself and want to pursue this more basic level of research, and gaining basic experience will be harder once training is complete.

3.2 Giving Talks

In training, and most likely in your professional life, you will be asked to give talks. There is an art to a well-done talk and having a reputation as a good speaker will serve you well throughout your career. You should not despair if you fear public speaking: good speakers are not born, they are made. Having given countless talks and having sat through many more, I have strong opinions about what makes a talk special. There are three criteria for an outstanding talk: (1) be useful and relevant; (2) include personal anecdotes; and (3) end a few minutes early.

3.2.1 Relevance: Consider the Audience

Making the talk useful and relevant is mandatory. Is there anything more irritating than attending a lecture that is clearly geared towards a different audience? Grand Rounds and resident noon conferences are difference venues with different purposes and audiences: a talk for one cannot be interchanged for another. A phrase you should never utter: "Oh, this slide is for a different audience, I'll skip it." If you find yourself thinking this as you run through your slides (see section on practice, later), fix the slide.

Think about what the audience needs to hear: exciting new advances in the field, bare-bones board review topics, or a case-based management tutorial? While it takes more time and energy to tailor talks to the audience, it's better than wasting the audience's time with a talk that won't help them.

There are faculty who elevate this practice to a fine art. I attended a Grand Rounds talk on acute heart failure. The speaker was from another institution and must have given that talk at least a hundred times in the preceding 25 years, yet she made it special. She included studies authored by faculty at my institution and highlighted the participation of those faculty members. At another Grand Rounds, the speaker began with a slide of the history of our medical center, highlighting the remarkable advances in cardiology at our institution over the past decade. In both cases, personalizing the talk for the audience took extra time and effort. By doing so, these speakers showed the audience that they held the institution in high regard: they made us feel as if they were talking only to us, and we were captivated.

3.2.2 The Importance of Anecdotes

A sense of humor is not mandatory, though an illustrative anecdote here or there (you will have more as you gain experience) is a wonderful way to connect with listeners. I give many talks on guideline-directed medical therapy in heart failure. I focus on sacubitril/valsartan as a game-changer. When the PARADIGM-HF trial came out in August 2014 (McMurray et al. 2014), it was the first time since the A-HeFT trial in 2004 (Taylor et al 2004) that a medication was shown to improve mortality in patients with heart failure.

I describe how exciting this was to a heart failure cardiologist at the time: I remember exactly where I was when the PARADIGM-HF trial was reported in August 2014 at the European Society of Cardiology meeting. I was at the airport, about to board a plane for the annual Kittleson family vacation to a lake house in Wisconsin. The *New England Journal of Medicine* Table of Contents appeared in my email with late-breaking trials from the ESC meeting. Seeing the PARADIGM-HF trial, I figured I'd read the abstract before we boarded as I expected it would be a disappointing negative trial like every other over the past decade. I would read it, sigh in despair, delete the email, and get on with my vacation.

Imagine my excitement when I saw the results: the first time since 2004 that a medication was shown to improve survival in heart failure and the first time since 1987 that any medication demonstrated superiority to an ACE inhibitor (Effects of enalapril on mortality in severe congestive heart failure 1987). I stood, transfixed by the survival curves on the iPhone screen, until my toddler's screeching broke my reverie: it was time to load the wild child onto the plane.

By sharing this anecdote of my own visceral reaction to this trial, I can impress upon the audience how pivotal sacubitril/valsartan is in the care of heart failure patients. Every so often, a talk I give is posted on YouTube and I know they make an impact. How? Both physicians and patients have asked me about the Kittleson family vacation when I recommend or prescribe sacubitril/valsartan.

The internet is also replete with pithy quotes and cartoons that may illustrate the point of your talk. Feel free to imitate others (with attribution, of course). If you hear a terrific talk, ask if you can borrow the slides with due credit provided. Anecdotes and humor promote effective learning.

3.2.3 Punctuality is a Virtue

Ending early is a wonderful bonus and ending late is never, ever okay. I have attended symposia where the program is running two hours late by the end of the day because speakers cannot adhere to the time limit. Sitting in the audience, gritting my teeth, I have fantasies about how conferences would run if I were in charge: microphones silenced when time was up, or vaudeville hooks emerging from the sidelines to pull inexperienced speakers offstage when the time limit is reached.

Don't inspire these fantasies in your audience. Ending a lecture late signals lack of respect for your audience (and the speakers following you if you're in the middle of a conference). If you cannot manage to cover the topic in the allotted time, then you are the problem, not the topic nor the time limit. No topic is so endlessly fascinating that people will forgive you for going over time. People have finite attention spans. Keep to the time limit.

3.2.4 Make Your Slides Work for You

Other phrases you should never utter during a talk: "Sorry the font is so small" or "Sorry this is a busy slide." Increase the font size. Put less on the slide. Make it simple. Use animation to highlight points rather than a laser pointer. Laser pointers are good for amusing cats but not much else. Waving a laser pointer around to punctuate your thoughts is a nervous tic that only serves to make your audience seasick. If you practice, you'll notice these problems and adjust the slides accordingly so when you're in front of the audience, your delivery is smooth and polished with not a queasy listener in the audience.

3.2.5 Practice, Practice, Practice

My magic formula is to practice a talk at least 7 times, timing myself, to ensure it is perfect. When a speaker appears natural and fluent, they are likely not a naturally gifted speaker. Rather, they have practiced (and practiced and practiced) the material to guarantee a smooth delivery.

I experienced a month of sleepless nights from anticipated dread when I had to give my first 10-minute oral abstract presentation at a national conference. I asked my mentor, who coached me through the presentation, if she became nervous before every talk. She said yes, of course, though the time she spent feeling nervous diminished over the years. As a trainee, she would endure many sleepless nights. As an experienced attending physician, she might have butterflies just before she began to speak. While I was doubtful at the time that I would ever approach a talk with her *sang froid*, it turns out she was right.

Put in the time and effort and energy—it will pay off, years later, when you can whip together custom slides perfectly pitched to the audience. You will practice to make it perfect within days, instead of weeks. You will be at ease because you will have experience borne of practice.

3.3 Choosing a Specialty

3.3.1 Process of Elimination

My counterintuitive take: choosing a specialty is a process of elimination. You must identify what does not appeal to you on the way to finding your passion. Medical students are like detectives. A detective narrows down the list of suspects to identify the perpetrator. Along the way, they eliminate the unlikely candidates through a mix of methodical plodding interspersed with flashes of inspiration and intuition. Just so, approach your search of specialty with an organized understanding of your strengths and priorities along with a mind open to possibility.

People often ask me why I chose to go into cardiology. I tell them the truth: it was a process of elimination. I knew surgery would never work; time in the operating room crawled; I was not enchanted by endless dissection. Obstetrics/gynecology was out for similar reasons, and because pregnancy scared me; the combination of limitless miracles and imminent disaster was too stressful. I ruled out radiology and pathology because I would miss patient interaction and psychiatry because I would miss the physical examination. So internal medicine was left standing: it was also the most practical and efficient use of all the knowledge I had painstakingly memorized in medical school and therefore the best fit for me. The first step in figuring out your specialty: figure out what you don't like. Is it clinics, intensive care units, operating rooms, dark rooms, microscopes?

3.3.2 What Do You Love?

When you've ruled out what will not work for you, you can then better figure out what does. For me, cardiology offered everything I loved: (1) the history and physical examination really make a difference (you cannot diagnose unstable angina without a history or decompensated heart failure without a physical examination); (2) there is a wide range of experience from inpatient, outpatient, and ICU-level care along with imaging and procedures; and (3) due to a rich decades-long history of randomized controlled trials, patients are offered therapies that work. This is not meant to be a commercial for a career in cardiology (though it's okay if I've convinced you that it's the best); rather, consider it a system for how to approach the array of specialties available to you.

3.3.3 Who Inspires You?

Besides process of elimination as a method to uncover your chosen specialty, mentors will also inspire you. I had great respect for many of my surgical attending physicians, including one who said that surgeons had to be internists first and surgeons second, as the key to surgery was to know when not to operate. Still, I knew I could never become him because I would be the surgeon who never wanted to operate.

Rather, it was an internist in medical school who inspired me. His ability to cogently translate the pathophysiology of a disease into etiology and thus differential diagnosis was extraordinary. I knew that if I could model myself after him, I would have a fulfilling career. We worked together for a few weeks and that's all it took. Identifying physicians who become inspiring role models—this is a wonderful way to choose a specialty.

Patients and family members can inspire you too. My grandfather had his first myocardial infarction at the age of 42, underwent coronary artery bypass surgery at 68 when I was in elementary school, and ultimately passed away from ischemic cardiomyopathy at the age of 85 when I was an internal medicine intern. His life was a triumph of medical care, borne of scientific advances and gifted physicians. While I grew up knowing he had coronary artery disease, it was only in medical school and residency that I understood the details of his care and grasped the miracle of his longevity. He passed away decades ago, yet I think he would be proud to know that one reason I chose heart failure as my specialty was to help other patients experience the same miracles he did.

3.3.4 Does Lifestyle Matter?

When I was in medical school, a common piece of advice was, "If you can think of anything you like better than surgery, do it," the assumption being that surgery was so taxing that it would require extraordinary dedication to withstand the rigors of training and the surgeon's lifestyle. This may be true for some types of surgery where cases can't be scheduled, emergencies are commonplace, and dedication even when not "on call" is critical to optimal patient care. Still, in some surgical subspecialties, flexibility is still possible. The specialty alone does not dictate the lifestyle. I know dermatologists who put in 16-hour days and cardiologists who work part-time on a predictable schedule.

While work-life balance is critical and should be one factor in your choice of specialty, it should not be the primary one. If you are concerned about what your life will look like if you choose a specialty you're passionate about, talk to physicians in that field. Seek out physicians in different types of practice environments within that field: academic, private practice large group, private practice small group, etc. You may find the lifestyle options are better than you thought—or not. Either way, you will enter the specialty with a better sense of what your future life in that specialty will hold.

3.3.5 What Comes Next

Once you've settled on a specialty, the next step is to fill your schedule with electives outside your specialty. When I decided that internal medicine was my passion in medical school, I did elective rotations in ophthalmology, radiology, and trauma surgery, realizing that I would never work in these fields again. When I identified cardiology as my specialty of choice as a resident, I filled my senior-year electives with oncology and the medical intensive care unit, figuring that I had the rest of my life to learn cardiology. And when I settled on a career as a heart failure/transplant cardiologist, I spent my final-year electives in the cardiac catheterization laboratory and in electrophysiology.

The knowledge you gain in rotations outside your chosen specialty will never be wasted; use every opportunity to gain experience.

3.4 Picking a Training Program

Once you've settled on a research versus clinical focus and chosen the specialty you love the most, you must critically evaluate training programs. As you hit the residency or fellowship interview trail, programs will start to blur together. Which one had night float and which one a call team? Which trainees rotated at three hospitals and which trainees rotated at two? These relatively minor details are not the dealbreakers; rather, you want to get a sense of the culture of various institutions and how the culture aligns with your ideal learning environment. The culture of medical education is best described by three tenets: volume, autonomy, and mentorship.

3.4.1 Volume

As Aristotle said, "We are what we repeatedly do. Excellence, then, is not an act, but a habit." And what is a habit but system of concrete action plans? This is true in medical education. The more you experience, the more you do, the better you become. Some learners enjoy a fast-paced, high-volume approach (drinking from a firehose). Others will learn better with a slower pace (sipping from a teacup) that allows time to deliberate and absorb. Know your style and judge programs accordingly by the volume of patients treated on various rotations.

For cardiology fellowship training programs in particular, you can ask how many beds are in the coronary care unit and are they always full? How many coronary angiograms will a fellow complete in a month-long rotation? How many heart transplants does the institution do annually? It is also useful to ask trainees where they feel there may be gaps in their training based on case volumes.

3.4.2   Autonomy

As discussed in the oral presentation section in Chap. 2, it's essential to be a captain, not a waiter: take ownership of the patient's management and you will learn. However, some learners do better with more autonomy to figure things out themselves while others prefer more support and supervision. I was the kind of resident who couldn't learn something if it was taught to me in a noon lecture. The role of vitamin D and parathyroid hormone in the evaluation of hypocalcemia was something I could dutifully memorize though I still had to look up before every examination. Then I admitted a patient to the hospital with numbness and tingling in her fingers and severe hypocalcemia. She was ultimately diagnosed with celiac sprue and the associated malabsorption resulted in vitamin D deficiency and thus hypocalcemia. Though I cared for this patient over two decades ago, I can still remember the physiology of vitamin D in calcium metabolism. Understanding my preferred learning style, I sought out a training program where autonomy would be prioritized. I knew I would learn best if I was expected to take ownership of my patients.

While the level of autonomy will be a relationship that each trainee negotiates with each attending physician based on the trainee's preference and the attending's style, programs generally have cultures of autonomy. The program's trainees can offer insight. Do senior medical residents run rounds? Do senior surgical residents perform the important parts of surgeries? Can senior residents perform procedures such as central lines and thoracenteses independently? Ultimately, does the culture of the program treat trainees like Captains, or like Waiters?

3.4.3   Mentorship

Mentorship is simply the ability to find role models who are willing to share their journey and advice with you (see the More About Mentors section later in the chapter). Ask trainees at various programs this: If you find an attending physician you want to be like when you grow up, are they open and willing to mentor you? You will need to seek out mentors; most need an encouraging nudge, a tap on the shoulder, a leading question. Once you show interest and make the effort to communicate, your effort will reap rewards. More on how to make the most of the mentor relationship next.

3.5   More About Mentors

You should have mentors throughout your career. Some you'll encounter through formal networking sessions where you are assigned to a faculty member in your training program. These always felt to me like well-intentioned, but awkward, blind dates where we both hesitated about whether we should commit to a second date. Other mentors you'll discover because you'll seek out connection with physicians who inspire you. The latter approach is my favorite: here's how you make the most of these intentional connections.

3.5.1   Find a Role Model

Mentor–mentee relationships more often (and perhaps more effectively) spring up organically. The only question you need ask yourself is: Who do I want to be like when I grow up? When you find that person, after working together on ward rotations or research projects, or after hearing them lecture, seek them out. Chances are, they will be flattered by your attention. If they are not, then they would have made a poor mentor anyway, and nothing is lost.

3.5.2   Ask the Right Questions

If you find a role model interested in being your mentor, and you're not sure where to go from there, the best question to ask is: How did you end up here? Nearly everyone loves talking about themselves so you will immediately forge a connection with the would-be mentor. In addition, learning how someone you admire, whose career successes appear impossibly out of reach, transformed their inexperience into experience will provide invaluable inspiration on how to navigate your career.

I was once in the cardiac catheterization laboratory waiting to start a case with another attending cardiologist waiting to start his. Killing time, I asked him how he ended up on faculty. What started as small talk turned into an inspiring story of serendipity. He recounted how, as a foreign medical graduate unsure of how he would obtain a residency position in the United States, he visited a friend who was a resident at a small hospital in the Midwest. The friend invited him on rounds and the attending physician was so impressed by the mysterious interloper's fund of knowledge and clinical judgment that she became his champion, pivotal in securing his residency position. With a foot in the door, my colleague quickly rose through the ranks and, decades later, he is a world-renowned cardiologist.

All at once, my feigned enthusiasm became real enthusiasm, and my colleague became my mentor. What struck me about his story was the element of chance: what if his friend hadn't invited him on rounds? There was also the element of preparation: my colleague used this opportunity to his advantage, shining based on his fund of knowledge borne of hard work. Louis Pasteur said, "Chance favors only the prepared mind". As I gather stories of the journeys of my mentors, a theme emerges: chance matters, and so does preparation. Start the conversation with any would-be mentor with the question: How did you end up here? You will learn so much from the answers.

3.5.3 Assemble a Cabinet

Think of mentors like your cabinet of advisors, each with a special area of expertise. Every kid knows that when you need to ask for permission, you ask Mom if you want a no and ask Dad if you want a yes. This is true for mentors too; each physician has a different style of practice. If you aren't sure if a patient needs to have an intervention, you'll ask a clinical mentor who's a minimalist and contrast the response with a mentor who's less conservative. If you have a question about the tips and tricks for nursing your baby at home and pumping at work, you'll know that some of your mentors will provide more useful answers than others.

There will also be the anti-role models, those you encounter who demonstrate behaviors you will be conscious not to emulate: the attending physician who ignores medical students, fails to make eye contact with patients, is always late to rounds. You will learn as much from bad behavior as good: be open to all opportunities for learning.

You will build your mentor cabinet over time as you make more connections at different levels of training. Some mentors will be with you for decades while others you may not ask for advice once you leave their local orbit. No one mentor can be all things to one mentee. Seek out research mentors, clinical mentors, administrative/leadership mentors, and work–life balance mentors as your career progresses.

3.6 Final Thoughts

Selecting research projects, giving talks, choosing your specialty, selecting training programs, finding mentors—navigating these areas successfully will serve you well in your career in medicine. Your medical career may follow one of many different paths, and the direction that brings you joy may change over time as you learn and grow. Use these skills to shine and provide optimal patient care no matter what direction your career heads.

References

Effects of enalapril on mortality in severe congestive heart failure. Results of the Cooperative North Scandinavian Enalapril Survival Study (CONSENSUS). The CONSENSUS Trial Study Group. N Engl J Med. 1987;316:1429–35.

Taylor AL, Ziesche S, Yancy C, Carson P, D'Agostino R, Ferdinand K, Taylor M, Adams K, Sabolinski M, Worcel M and Cohn JN. Combination of isosorbide dinitrate and hydralazine in blacks with heart failure. N Engl J Med. 2004;351:2049–57.

McMurray JJ, Packer M, Desai AS, Gong J, Lefkowitz MP, Rizkala AR, Rouleau JL, Shi VC, Solomon SD, Swedberg K, Zile MR, Investigators P-H and Committees. Angiotensin-neprilysin inhibition versus enalapril in heart failure. N Engl J Med. 2014;371:993–1004.

Part II
Honing Your Clinical Judgment

Chapter 4
Diagnosis

There are many difficult and steep learning curves in the transition from the didactic years of medical school to the clinical ones. One particular challenge is mastering the art of differential diagnosis. Reading textbooks is easy: each disease is presented in an orderly fashion, described by its history, physical examination, laboratory findings, and management. However, patients don't present with diseases, they present with symptoms. An experienced physician knows how to work backwards, organizing the symptoms into a list of likely diseases that could be causing them. This art, of differential diagnosis, is a talent that takes years of experience to master.

As a fledgling clinician, however, you don't have years to master the art of differential diagnosis. Sir William Osler said, "Medicine is a science of uncertainty and an art of probability" and this aphorism sums up differential diagnosis in a nutshell. An inexperienced clinician can list 17 causes of chest discomfort. An experienced clinician can easily, almost unconsciously, rank this list based on the patient's risk factors and presentation and what's common, such that costochondritis and aortic dissection and mediastinal masses do not receive the same serious consideration.

There are medical strategies to aid in differential diagnosis. The first step begins in medical school where you take on the painstaking task of memorizing the grammar and vocabulary of medicine (described in Chap. 1) so you can later string those facts together to fluently appreciate the poetry of differential diagnosis. Once you have established the foundation of facts, the next step is to move away from rote memorization into medical reasoning: etiology flows naturally from pathophysiology.

If a patient has edema, you will remember that the pathophysiology of edema involves an increase in hydrostatic pressure or a decrease in oncotic pressure. You will organize the conditions that increase hydrostatic pressure as a global increase in volume from heart failure or renal failure and a local increase from obstruction in venous return from pregnancy, obesity, or deep vein thrombosis. You will then organize the conditions that decreased oncotic pressure as those that involve decreased protein production such as malnutrition and liver disease and those that involve increased protein loss such as nephrotic syndrome. Just like that, you will have identified eight broad categories of causes of edema which you can then subdivide further: is the heart failure related to a problem with the heart muscle, valves, arteries, or pericardium, and so on. Just like that—the rote memorization that aided you in the early years of medical school is transformed into the poetry of medical reasoning.

The second strategy to aid in differential diagnosis is to separate those diagnoses that are serious from those that are benign. Even if you believe that aortic dissection is less likely than costochondritis in a patient presenting with chest pain, you must be satisfied that you have done the medical due diligence to exclude aortic dissection. This does not mean that every patient with chest pain needs a chest CT. Rather, always remember the serious, dangerous, life-threatening causes and perform a directed history and physical examination that either excludes those causes or indicates the need for further investigation.

What about the general approaches to honing your clinical acumen? Here are some of the approaches that experienced clinicians use to figure out the likely disease behind the symptoms.

4.1   Read a Lot (of Notes)

As an early career physician, when I would round on my colleagues' patients in the hospital on the weekend, I would read the charts—and not just the notes from the current hospitalization. I would read notes from prior clinic visits and hospitalizations. I did this because I was curious about each patients' illness story: how did they present, how long did it take to make the diagnosis, what clues might there have been to the diagnosis before it was discovered, what was the highest-yield testing that uncovered the diagnosis, and so forth.

Rounding one weekend, I fell down the rabbit hole of a fascinating case. A middle-aged woman presented with heart failure and severe aortic regurgitation and underwent aortic valve replacement. Intraoperatively, she was noted to have evidence of inflammation of the aorta and elevated serum inflammatory markers as well as elevated beta-D-glucan, a marker of fungal infection. Even though she didn't appear sick enough to have a fungal endocarditis, and the valve pathology itself showed no inflammation, she received a course antifungal therapy.

Two years later, her shortness of breath returned, and an echocardiogram showed severe paravalvular aortic regurgitation and a dilated aortic root. She underwent redo aortic valve replacement and reduction aortoplasty. Curiously, this time an aortic root abscess was noted intraoperatively and pathology consistent with inflammation and organized vegetation. Cultures were negative but she was treated empirically with vancomycin/ceftriaxone for 6 weeks.

It wasn't until a year later, when she presented with joint pain and was referred to a rheumatologist that the diagnosis was finally made. A CT scan of the chest showed an inflammatory process affecting the aortic arch and left subclavian artery most consistent with Takayasu's arteritis. Despite treatment with immunosuppressive therapy, she again developed severe aortic regurgitation; by this point, she was not a candidate for a third aortic valve replacement and warranted evaluation for heart transplantation.

Takayasu's arteritis is a difficult diagnosis to make. In this case, the clues were there: inflammation of the aorta but not the aortic valve with no evidence of infection—in retrospect, the presence of a large-vessel vasculitis can seem obvious. The better question is: what could the treating physicians at the time done differently?

I made a mental list of all the places where the story didn't make sense: why would a middle-aged woman with a structurally normal aortic valve develop aortic regurgitation in the first place? Why would she have inflammation of the aorta with no signs of infection at the time of not just the first, but also the second, surgery? Why would the first valve replacement fail within a few years with no evidence of infection as a cause? Hindsight is 20/20 and the goal is not Monday-morning quarterbacking. Rather, the goal is to gain the same experience as the treating physicians did when they finally made this rare diagnosis and all the pieces fell into place.

If those physicians who treated this patient ever encountered another patient with an intraoperative aortitis, they would have vasculitis on their differential. By doing a deep dive into the chart of a patient with an unusual diagnosis, you too can gain experience even though you haven't care for the patient firsthand.

Make this a habit. When you uncover a patient with an unusual diagnosis, do a chart dive: explore the presenting symptoms. If there are delays in diagnosis, challenge yourself to identify potentially missed clinical clues or pitfalls of the tests ordered. Use every bit of information at your disposal to gain valuable experience. Your colleagues can be your mentors—even through their notes.

4.2 The Highest-Yield Questions

Experienced clinicians know the best questions to ask patients to figure out the most important answers: sick or not sick, and what's the diagnosis. Of all the questions one can ask a patient to determine the cause of their symptoms, the ones I find the highest yield are.

4.2.1 What Are the Precipitating, Exacerbating, and Relieving Factors?

You may ask why the nature of the symptom is not included here. Sometimes, the description of the pain itself can be misleading. I once saw a patient with shortness of breath. He had sought out evaluation with one of his college roommates who happened to be a pulmonologist, convinced that he had asthma. The pulmonologist heard the story of progressive exertional dyspnea relieved by rest and walked the patient across the hall to my cardiology office. A stress echocardiogram reproduced symptoms at a low level of exertion with multiple wall motion abnormalities consistent with multi-vessel coronary disease. He had an angiogram a few days later followed by bypass surgery. What was the clue here? It was not the nature of the symptom—it was the context.

In Boston, chest pain may be "wicked shaaahp" when it's not sharp or stabbing at all, just severe. And patients with angina will often correct you when you inquire about pain: "It's not a pain, it's a pressure." Angina can also be a burning or aching discomfort, nausea, or shortness of breath. The old truism that any symptom from the nose to the navel can be angina is correct. The important distinction, however, is in the triggers which tend to be universal and reliable, and offer insight into the story of the presentation.

4.2.2   Have the Symptoms Been Getting Better, Worse, or Staying the Same and Over What Period of Time?

Patient's symptoms have a trajectory and patient stories have a rhythm. Symptoms get better, or get worse, or wax and wane, or have periods of calm punctuated by intense exacerbations. Have the palpitations been going on for 10 years, occurring three nights a week right before bed for a few seconds, triggered mainly by drinking wine with dinner? Probably benign premature beats. Does the heart race abruptly for minutes accompanied by near-fainting and, over the past week, shortness of breath? Maybe a re-entrant tachycardia with cardiomyopathy. If you are willing to ask enough questions, know the alarm symptoms, and are able direct testing accordingly, you will find the answer.

A patient came to see me for evaluation of seizures, an unusual indication for a cardiology consultation. However, on listening to her story, I was grateful that her cousin, a surgical colleague, encouraged her to see me. She described seizures that were preceded by lightheadedness and nausea. Her neurological evaluation was normal, and she was told that she would need seizure medications for life. Then she confessed another symptom, telling me she felt weird even mentioning it because she knew it sounded crazy: she could feel her heart slowing down as if it were going to stop before each episode.

Her symptoms were severe and recurrent, so I dug deeper. An ambulatory ECG monitor was unrevealing, and I remained undeterred. It's important to know the pitfalls of the tests you order (more on this in Chap. 5). In this case, it was the fact that she had no symptoms while wearing the ambulatory ECG monitor—a monitor is only "negative" or "normal" if there are no arrhythmias noted during symptoms. If the patient has no symptoms while wearing the monitor, then the test is inadequate. Because I was concerned that there was something more concerning than anxiety afoot, I ordered a tilt table test to see if she had severe vasovagal syncope.

Lo and behold, it reproduced her symptoms—with a vengeance. She had asystole for 30 s requiring atropine and transcutaneous pacing. It was the severe vasovagal syncope that caused hypoperfusion and subsequent seizure activity. The electrophysiologist monitoring the test called me to report the findings and his first words were, "Thanks—but I didn't need any more gray hairs." When I went to see her in the recovery area, her first words were also "Thank you," followed by something I'll never forget. She said, "I feel vindicated." She had a pacemaker placed and stopped taking antiseizure medications. Now, over a decade later, she has never had another episode though she will feel herself pacing from time to time.

What's the lesson here? Listen to the patient. Dramatic, severe, worsening symptoms require a more careful look. We all know that the longer a symptom has been going on for, the less likely it is to be life-threatening. The caveat to this is worsening symptoms. A symptom that progresses should be respected, investigated, and understood.

4.2.3 What Made You Decide to Come in Today to Discuss Your Symptoms?

Sometimes a patient has had a symptom forever and something triggers them to seek medical attention. When the trajectory is flat but the patient is concerned, the trigger can offer insight. I once saw multiple members of the same religious congregation for cardiac evaluations within a span of a few months. It was not until a grieving mother came to see me that I discovered the source of the flurry of consultations. Her young daughter, a member of the congregation, had been diagnosed with peripartum cardiomyopathy and, shortly thereafter, died in her sleep. In this case, there was nothing contagious or hereditary in her devastating and tragic death. Her family, friends, and members of the congregation did not have a medical basis for their fear and desire for cardiac evaluations. However, knowing the impetus for the rush of cardiac evaluations helped me better evaluate, counsel, and reassure the patients.

When the impetus is not clear, probe. Was their next-door neighbor with the same symptoms just diagnosed with cancer? Did a friend prod them to finally seek medical attention? Or is the symptom now interfering with their activities? Did they uncover a scary diagnosis on Dr. Google? Knowing the trigger may help differentiate between anxiety and something serious.

4.2.4 What Are You Most Worried About?

My father, an internist in private practice for decades, used to sit at the dining table after supper and call his patients to relay lab results. No electronic medical records or nurse to field calls—just a stack of paper charts, a felt-tip pen, his photographic memory for hundreds of phone numbers, and meticulous handwritten notes. Sometimes, I heard him say, "Well, what do you think it is?" I would joke with him: wasn't it his job, as the doctor, to tell the patient what the diagnosis was? Now, as a physician, I see the value in this question.

First, there may be insight into the true diagnosis: is the patient worried about shortness of breath because his mother and two cousins passed away from heart failure, signaling a possible familial cardiomyopathy or inherited arrhythmia syndrome?

Second, obtaining insight into the patient's true fears allows you to alleviate them most effectively. I saw a patient once with palpitations from symptomatic PVCs documented on ambulatory ECG monitoring. She was convinced that she had atrial fibrillation and when pressed, admitted that she was terrified of having a stroke, like her elderly father who had atrial fibrillation. Though this was not her diagnosis, better understanding her fear helped me clearly explain how her father's history was distinct from hers and why she was at low risk for stroke. She wasn't really worried about atrial fibrillation; she was grieving the transformation of her robust father into an invalid. Understanding her fears allowed me to help her best.

Finally, the source of a patient's concerns may offer other ways to help them. When I was a cardiology fellow, a patient came to clinic after every dental cleaning requesting an echocardiogram to exclude infective endocarditis. She has no personal or family history of this, and no risk factors. Infective endocarditis turned out to be just one of her many worries. Instead of ordering an echocardiogram and sending her on her way (the quick and painless route), my cardiology attending physician took the time to talk to her about her anxiety.

My attending physician helped the patient realize that the treatment for her anxiety was not an echocardiogram; the best treatment was establishing care with a therapist. By the end of the visit, the patient thanked my attending physician for talking to her rather than at her and gave her a hug. That moment has stayed with me: sometimes giving the patient what they need is different from giving them what they want; the art of medicine is charting the diagnostic and management plan together. Although this case turned out well, my attending's efforts could have backfired. The patient could have been resistant and insulted and delivered a scathing anonymous review (more on these reviews in Chap. 13).

4.2.5 *What Have You Tried to Make It Better? What Prior Testing Have You Had?*

Learn from the past. Often, you will not be the first physician encounter for a patient with a given symptom. Knowing what has been tried and worked or failed, and what prior testing has revealed, will allow you to seamlessly take over the patient's care instead of performing redundant, unnecessary, and often costly investigations. The former approach inspires trust. The latter can delay appropriate care.

Knowing a patient with a lingering upper respiratory infection has already been given azithromycin and levofloxacin with little effect will help you convince them that a third course of antibiotics directed at what is likely a viral illness will be unsuccessful. Knowing that a patient with heart failure has already undergone testing for HIV, ferritin, and TSH allows you to avoid unneeded testing as you investigate potential causes for their nonischemic cardiomyopathy.

4.3   Learning More Than What the Patient Says

There are times when I miss a diagnosis. Of course, no one's perfect, but the stakes are high in cardiology. When this happens, I go back and review where I went wrong. At times, it's because I failed to ask the key high-yield questions. Other times, it's because I failed to hear more than what the patient was saying. I cared for an elderly woman with severe aortic stenosis who underwent transcatheter aortic valve replacement (TAVR). The pre-procedure coronary angiogram showed no coronary artery disease and the echocardiogram post TAVR was perfect.

However, a few months later, she reported arm pain. It was odd, and specific: if she used her arms too much when folding clothes, they would feel achy and the pain only improved if she rested and drank cold water. She came back a few more times over the next few months with the same symptoms, and I reassured her that her pain was not cardiac because her symptoms were not triggered with exertion and were stable, and because she had a normal angiogram just a few months prior.

Then, her husband passed away, and she presented with shortness of breath. Echocardiogram showed an ejection fraction of 25% with apical ballooning consistent with a stress cardiomyopathy. Since stress cardiomyopathy is a diagnosis of exclusion, she underwent coronary angiography which showed a new 99% ostial left main stenosis that appeared mechanical and related to TAVR placement. This is a zebra of a diagnosis with just a few case reports in the literature. I missed this rare diagnosis even though I had considered all the high-yield questions. What did I miss? I missed listening to more than what the patient was saying to me.

For this patient, there is a happy ending. Her left main stent went in without a hitch, her ejection fraction normalized, and she went back to shuttling the grandkids to afterschool activities. But I still think about this close call and the lessons I have learned to prevent it from happening to another patient.

4.3.1   Personality

Some patients will report every symptom to you, while others mention nothing unless prodded. This patient fell into the latter category. I should have realized that it was not in her nature return for multiple visits after I had already reassured her. When a patient presents more than once with the same symptom, the subsequent evaluation needs to be more detailed than the original one. I should have delved more deeply into the source of her symptoms.

4.3.2 Other Opinions

Family members can be a great resource. Some patients are minimizers and only their loved ones will tell you what's truly going on. Speaking to this patient's daughter after the fact, it turns out her symptoms were absolutely exertional, though the patient for did not report them as such.

4.3.3 Location

Most people dislike the emergency department. It's noisy and chaotic, and you have to wait a really long time to see a doctor. So a patient who doesn't call their doctor's office for an appointment, or go to urgent care, and goes to the ED instead, is a really worried patient. Every doctor takes a patient's symptoms more seriously when they show up to the ED. If a 60-year-old man has burning chest pain after dinner and presents to the ED that night and not to your office a week later, it probably means he needs more than a proton pump inhibitor.

4.3.4 Your (the Physician's) State of Mind

So many colleagues describe the difficulty of focusing on the patient in the room when faced with competing distractors in their head: they may be running 30 min behind; they may have forgotten to drop off their kid's art project at school; their manuscript might have been rejected on the second try; they may feel the existential dread of the pandemic bearing down on them, every minute of every day.

With experience, you can learn to control the distractors. If you're about to go into an exam room, and you're feeling frazzled because there are three other patients standing outside their exam rooms looking impatient, take a deep breath and remember that this is your inexperience talking. Remember what Maya Angelou once said, "I've learned that people will forget what you said, people will forget what you did, but people will never forget how you made them feel."

I asked a mentor once how she put her game face on and focused on her patients, no matter what else was going on in her life. She said something I'll never forget: For a physician, the patient encounter begins when they walk in the exam room. For a patient, the physician encounter begins when they call for the appointment, arrange time off from work, try to find parking at the medical center, sit in the waiting room, and wait in the exam room. For the patient, the moment when the physician walks in the exam room is a culmination of the effort it took to seek out care.

Experienced physicians see 20 clinic patients in a day and know that each patient will only see one doctor. This mentor advised me: if you feel like stifling a sigh when you're on visit 15 of 20, don't think of patients in terms of numbers standing between you and a break. Rather, think of them as people with problems who put in significant time and effort to see you. Remember how it feels to be the patient.

For a patient, even a routine visit is filled with anticipation and stress. One visit in a long string of visits for the physician may be the patient's event of the day. If you remember this, it will be easier to give patients your full attention and concentration. If you do this, you will be less likely to miss critical information. This focus will also make the visit more of a pleasure for you, and for them.

4.4 Diagnostic Pitfalls

Sometimes when you ask a patient a question, they answer a different one. Here are a few examples of making sure you and the patient are on the same page.

4.4.1 Orthopnea

If you ask a patient with heart failure if they feel short of breath when lying flat in bed, and they respond that they always sleep on two pillows, the conclusion is not that they have two-pillow orthopnea. Instead, delve deeper: are those two pillows for comfort, or for breathing? Sleeping on two pillows is not two-pillow orthopnea unless the patient would be too short of breath to sleep without the two pillows. Understand patients completely: in our line of work, lives depend on it.

4.4.2 Reproducible Chest Pain

If a patient presents with chest pain and says, "Ouch," when you press on the left fourth costochondral junction, this doesn't mean the patient has costochondritis. Rather, the patient may have musculoskeletal strain in addition to angina. An important follow-up question is, "Does this tenderness I'm eliciting with pressure resemble the discomfort that brought you in today?" Eliciting pain on palpation is not a free pass to cross angina off your differential diagnosis. Use context and triggers to narrow in on the source.

4.4.3 Assessment of Mental Status

When I was young and inexperienced, I diagnosed a patient with a stroke because of slurred speech, only to discover that she was not wearing her dentures. Once in, her speech was perfect. (In fact, the neurology resident called for the stat consultation was not amused when the patient put in her dentures, sipped some water, and proudly recited "She sells seashells by the seashore" five times in a row, more fluently that I could have. I still wince, my pride smarting, whenever I hear that tongue twister.)

Yes, this example is funny, and I'm the punchline. It's also serious. The patient was subjected to an urgent neurologic evaluation that panicked both her and her family. I summoned the neurology resident unnecessarily and this might have delayed the care of other patients with true neurologic emergencies. What's the lesson here? Know your patient. Details matter: when assessing mental status, make sure the patient speaks your language and has their glasses, hearing aids, and dentures in place to make it a fair evaluation.

4.5 The Power of Observation

Physicians stake their reputation on their powers of observation. Interacting with person after person, asking questions and absorbing responses, convincing, cajoling, elaborating, explaining; the experienced clinician gains an unconscious sense of which patient is buying what they're selling and which patient is not. Aside from tells and microexpressions, there are several observational skills that will serve you well before you ask even one of the high-yield diagnostic questions.

4.5.1 Walking in the Exam Room

If you happen to be lingering in the hallway of clinic, you may observe your patient as the nurse brings them into the exam room. Are they stooped and shuffling, stopping due to shortness of breath, unsteady on their feet? Already, you have a sense of their strength, conditioning, and overall health.

4.5.2 Who's with the Patient?

Caregivers, family, and accompanying friends can tell you a lot. The first question is, who's there, or not there? I cared for a young man with advanced heart failure. His mother was at his bedside in the intensive care unit for the months he spent waiting for a new heart and the months he spent recovering from a rocky post-operative course. When he was finally discharged, she faithfully drove him to every clinic appointment.

Imagine my surprise when, about a year after transplant, I walked into the exam room to see him, and his mother wasn't there. That's when I knew he was doing great—when his mother finally felt comfortable enough to let him come to an appointment alone. Turns out her instinct, borne of hours spent caring for him, was right—he was doing great. On the other hand, if there is no one with the patient and the patient is doing worse, ask yourself if the loss of support is responsible for this turn of events.

The converse is also true: when a patient who comes to every appointment independently now brings someone, something is amiss. The loved one may have accompanied the patient because they are concerned about a symptom and don't trust the patient to give the full story, or because the patient is worried about a symptom and has brought moral support. It may be that the patient can no longer care for themselves independently and now needs a caregiver for appointments, a sign of early dementia or debility.

When visitors are present, pay attention to the mood. Were there arguments, tension cut short abruptly as you opened the door? This bears investigation: is the patient's illness the source of stress or is the tension in the household contributing to the patient's symptoms, or both? Did laughter spill out as you walked in? Does it feel as if you entered the room in the middle of someone telling a joke at a party? The fun may be borne of nerves, though I find that patients and family members who are joking around in the exam room while waiting for the doctor are generally relaxed and the patient is doing well.

Finally, what is the visitor's attitude? Is it an attentive caregiver with notebook and pen in hand, or a disinterested mode of transplantation, glued only to their phone? That can give you a sense of what support the patient may have at home.

4.5.3   The Hospital Set-Up

For hospitalized patients, seeing who visits and when can be revealing. Nurses, at the bedside for 8–12 h shifts, are a great resource. The patient's bedside tray is also a rich source of insight into their health. Potato chips and Gatorade at the bedside of a patient admitted for heart failure means more education on dietary indiscretion triggering heart failure exacerbations is required. Is there a new paperback where before there was none? The patient is feeling better. Are there cards and flowers, or none at all? That can tell you what support the patient has from family and friends, or what financial stress those family and friends are under if there are no gifts at the bedside. It could be anything—the point is, pay attention and be aware of what's going on with your patients.

I cared for a patient awaiting heart transplantation. The walls of his room were plastered with photos of a cabin the woods. Turns out he had built the cabin himself and he hadn't been there in months because he was too sick to handle the altitude. How amazing that within 6 months of his transplant, he was back, chopping wood and doing repairs. The photos of him, catching fish in the nearby river, meant so much more to me because I knew what this milestone meant to him.

Learn as much as you can from the patient before you even talk to them: from their walk, from the company they bring to appointments, from the accoutrements on their bedside tray. All this information can help you place what they say into context that allows you to know the person and better understand their diagnosis. Diseases may become routine with experience; patients must not.

4.6   Final Thoughts

The adage goes, "The generalist knows nothing about everything and the specialist knows everything about nothing," Perhaps more accurate: "The generalist knows to diagnose and the specialist knows to treat." This is a generalization, of course—all experienced physicians should be great diagnosticians. The art of medicine begins with the art of the diagnosis. It is most important to know how to arrive at the right diagnosis, because then you will know how to direct your investigation into the best treatment strategy.

Chapter 5
Tests and Interventions

5.1 There is No Perfect Test

What is every doctor's dream? A test that tells you who is sick, who is not sick, and does so with 100% certainty. At the start of medical school, you think that every test operates this way. You're a third-year medical student on an internal medicine rotation, and you admit a patient with chest pain. Serial troponins are negative, so you order a stress test which is also negative, and you send the patient home, secure in the knowledge that you did a great job, and he is fine.

But is he? Does a negative troponin exclude critical coronary artery disease? I cared for a patient with a 2-month history of chest discomfort that occurred when he walked up hills while playing golf. It progressed to the point that he stopped playing golf and had to ask his wife to roll the trash cans out to the end of his driveway. He finally sought medical attention when he had discomfort walking up his front steps that wouldn't go away. In the ED, he appeared mildly anxious though pain-free. His EKG was normal. His troponin was negative. Still, I arranged for an urgent cardiac catheterization, on a Saturday afternoon, because his story was scary. What drove me to summon the weekend call team based only on a history, without confirmation from objective testing from the EKG or lab tests? I recognized the concerning trajectory of his symptoms and the pitfalls of the normal test results. Fortunately for this patient, by the time I met him, I had crossed the bridge from inexperience to experience.

I'll never forget his angiogram. As I engaged the right coronary artery and injected contrast, there was an oval lucency at the ostium of the right coronary artery, teetering in, teetering out, and causing progressive symptoms that might have ended in a large inferolateral myocardial infarction—but didn't.

What about an abnormal stress test? Does this exclude critical coronary artery disease? Every cardiologist, including me, will tell you the story of a patient with a good story and a negative stress test who is admitted to the hospital shortly after the negative stress test—with a myocardial infarction. Maybe the images on stress echocardiogram were technically limited. Maybe the patient had balanced ischemia on myocardial perfusion imaging such that reversible defects from ischemia were not appreciated. Maybe the patient did not achieve target heart rate, making it a nondiagnostic (rather than negative) test. The interpretation of a test starts with the patient: if your suspicion of coronary disease based on their history and other medical problems remains high, if you still have lingering doubt after a normal test result, it is essential to delve deeper to convince yourself it was a true negative. In other words, Bayes Theorem is your friend.

5.2 Bayes Theorem is Your Friend

The point here is not to know the pitfalls of every diagnostic test (more on this later in the chapter), but to realize that no test is perfect, and that every test result must be interpreted through the lens of your patient's history and physical examination. It is the history and physical examination that sets your pretest probability, and the purpose of the tests is not to discover the diagnosis, but to confirm or deny the suspected diagnosis based on the history and physical examination.

There are many reasons not to order a test: (1) you "just want to know" what it shows; (2) you already know what is shows; or (3) you don't care what it shows (because you already have a plan in place). Say you evaluate a young woman with chest pain every time she eats chili though she runs marathons without limitations. You "just want to be sure" so you order a stress test. It comes back abnormal, with ischemia in the anterior wall. Because your pre-test probability of coronary artery disease is low, the positive test doesn't change much: the chance of a false-positive is higher than the chance of a true-positive. What's more, you now have to explain to the patient why you are ignoring an abnormal result of a test you ordered, which erodes your credibility and the patient's confidence in you. Even worse, unnecessary tests will result in stress, anxiety, discomfort, and potential risk for the patient which must be avoided at all costs.

Unnecessary tests violate the overarching tenet of medicine, "First, do no harm," and sometimes at great cost to the patient. I cared for a young woman with an ischemic cardiomyopathy—and not from coronary artery disease. She reported chest pain to her internist who ordered a stress test which was abnormal. The internist referred her to a cardiologist who decided to perform a coronary angiogram. On angiogram, her coronary arteries were perfectly normal (no surprise, as her chest pain was not suggestive of coronary disease)—until she had an iatrogenic dissection of her left main coronary artery during the angiogram. She underwent emergency coronary artery bypass surgery and was left with an ischemic cardiomyopathy. Years later, she worsened and required heart transplantation with a difficult post-transplant course. *Iatrogenesis imperfecta*: she endured a terrible odyssey, precipitated by acting on a test that she never needed in the first place.

So, whenever you're thinking of ordering a test, do a thought experiment: what is your plan for a positive, negative, and indeterminate result? If the plan is the same regardless of the result, don't order the test. If you don't know what the plan should be for every possible result, you should not be ordering the test. The plan does not have to be exact; you don't need to know the specific management plan for every diagnosis you consider, from pheochromocytoma to Familial Mediterranean fever to chronic thromboembolic pulmonary hypertension. However, you do need to have a clear idea of the next step, whether it is confirmatory diagnosis testing or help from the appropriate consultant.

There are situations where a thought experiment will demonstrate that a test is not indicated. Consider a patient with a longstanding cardiomyopathy with a severely reduced ejection fraction and a severely dilated ventricle who is in cardiogenic shock and stabilized with inotropic support. The best option for such a patient to improve quality of life and survival is heart transplantation. However, during your investigation, you determine that the patient has never had a coronary angiogram to assess for ischemic heart disease as the source of the cardiomyopathy. While an evaluation for ischemia is standard in a patient with a newly diagnosed cardiomyopathy, especially in a patient with cardiac risk factors, the question is how an angiogram would impact the care of this patient with advanced heart failure in cardiogenic shock. If there were severe coronary artery disease amenable to revascularization, would that alter the patient's course and obviate the need for transplantation? The answer may be no and if so, the angiogram should not be performed.

5.3 Pitfalls, Outliers, and Trends

While you cannot know the pitfalls of every diagnostic test, every test has them and for the tests you order most often, you will learn the pitfalls with experience. As noted above, a stress test may show no ischemia because it is truly negative (there is no ischemia) or because the test was inadequate (technically limited images or inability to reach target heart rate). An ambulatory ECG monitor may uncover no arrhythmias because there are no arrhythmias causing the patient's symptoms of palpitations, or because the patient happened to have no symptoms while wearing the monitor. Other classic pitfalls: a normal uric acid level does not rule out gout, a positive D-dimer is not indicative of pulmonary embolism (because a D-dimer is sensitive for pulmonary embolism but not specific), and you can have unstable angina with a negative troponin.

Also not every abnormal laboratory finding is a cause for alarm. Mild abnormalities, especially in a patient who looks and feels well, may be outliers instead of trends. How do you decide if an abnormal result is an outlier or a trend? Consider how the patient looks/feels, the contribution of medical conditions to explain the finding, and how abnormal the result is. For example, if a patient on no medications who feels well has an elevated potassium of 5.8 mEq/L, it's reasonable to assume an outlier and repeat the test. On the other hand, if a patient who feels fatigued and nauseous has a potassium of 6.4 mEq/L and takes lisinopril and spironolactone, it is important to stop offending agents, prescribe a potassium-binder, and recheck within a few days.

5.4 Duplication of Effort

As a resident, every patient admitted with heart failure received an echocardiogram on admission. It didn't matter whether an echocardiogram had been done two days prior at another hospital prior to transfer—it was standard practice to obtain our *own* echocardiogram. While it's fantastic to review primary data rather than a report on paper, unnecessary testing is wasteful and puts patients through tests they don't need.

In the current era of immediate accessibility, request CDs for your imaging studies, upload them onto your hospital's imaging systems, and have them over-read if you feel necessary. Save the patient and the healthcare system the unnecessary step of extra testing. A small bit of effort on your part can make a big difference that patients will appreciate.

5.5 Communicate the Urgency

A family friend saw her internist for a routine check-up. The internist heard a murmur and ordered an echocardiogram that was scheduled to happen 3 weeks later. My friend was terrified: was her heart a ticking time bomb, did she need heart surgery, or was it okay to exercise and go on a planned family vacation to Bermuda later that month? After 2 weeks of sleepless nights, she broke down and called me for advice. Because she had no symptoms, the echocardiogram was not urgent, and it was perfectly fine to live her life with no restrictions or concerns during the medically appropriate 3-week wait for the echocardiogram. I explained that even if there was a valvular abnormality responsible for the murmur, her lack of symptoms suggested that the management probably would entail little more than follow-up echocardiograms every few years. She cried in relief, and it made me realize: a minor test to a physician may be misconstrued by the patient as the prelude to a life-threatening diagnosis.

I had been in the position of this inexperienced physician before, ordering a test without communicating the urgency to the patient. My friend's reaction was a clear demonstration for me of the consequences of this inexperience. When you order a test, the first step as described above is to do the thought experiment to confirm that it will change your management and you have a plan for every anticipated result. The next step is to communicate the urgency to the patient. What will the test entail, how urgently does the test need to be performed, and how long will it take to get the results? Patients need to know because they will be consumed by the unknowns. Maybe you know that, medically, it's fine if the test takes a week to happen, or a month—make sure they do too.

5.5.1 Prepare the Patient

Sometimes the responsibility to follow up on planned testing falls on you, even though it doesn't originate with you. I cared for a patient with hypertension and dyslipidemia. She didn't really need to a see a cardiologist routinely, but her internist had referred her years earlier so that I could convince her to take a statin and she saw me annually thereafter; she told me she liked the comfort and security of knowing she had a cardiologist in her medical orbit just in case.

She presented to the hospital one weekend with chest discomfort with a normal ECG and negative cardiac enzymes. Given her risk factors, a nuclear stress test was performed which showed a 3% reversible inferior defect most consistent with artifact. The cardiologist interpreting the study recommended a coronary CT angiogram (CCTA) for reassurance. She was discharged home over the weekend and told to follow up with me to schedule the CCTA.

Now, one could argue whether a patient with resolved chest pain not consistent with angina by history and no evidence of myocardial infarction and a low-risk stress test finding needed a CCTA, but given that the seed had been planted, I asked my assistant to arrange the study as requested. When my assistant called the patient to put the plan in motion, the patient was frantic. No one had explained to her prior to discharge that she needed another heart test, or why, and she did not understand why she had been discharged if her heart wasn't okay; she told my assistant that she was going to head right back to the hospital.

Once I called her and explained that the CCTA was to be performed in an (over)abundance of caution, that there was no urgency because she had no evidence of a heart attack, and that the results would help adjust medications (such as potential intensification of statin therapy), she was relieved. She was perfectly fine to wait a week for the next available CCTA appointment and to see me a few days later to go over the results. She was not unreasonable, just scared, and a little explanation went a long way to alleviating her fears.

5.5.2 The Acute Recognition of a Chronic Problem is not the Same as an Acute Problem

Imagine my family friend with the murmur presented to you for routine evaluation and you ordered the echocardiogram. Imagine that instead of suffering in silence about the 3-week delay in obtaining the echocardiogram, she requests that the echocardiogram be done immediately. You know that when the patient otherwise feels well, chances are the murmur has been present for a while, and the acute recognition of a chronic problem does not constitute an emergency. In this situation, stick to a medically appropriate, not patient-directed, timeline. The acute recognition of a chronic problem is not the same as an acute problem.

It is understandable that when a patient receives a diagnosis, they are scared and want that the problem be taken care of *yesterday*. This misplaced sense of urgency may stem from an inexperienced referring physician providing an inappropriate sense of urgency or not explaining the appropriate urgency so that the patient assumes the worst. Calibrate the urgency by whether the patient has an acute problem or a chronic problem, and don't confuse an acute problem for the acute recognition of a chronic problem.

Let the patient know why you are not pushing for an urgent appointment. Sometimes, patients ask me to advocate for a test ASAP when this is not medically indicated. I explain to them that I will not, because I respect the specialist who performs the test, and I need to reserve my urgent demands for cases of true medical urgency. Usually, patients are relieved to hear that they are not the emergency and are reassured that I have their best interest at heart: a win–win for communication and trust. The "I want it because I want it" culture serves no one in medicine—not physicians and certainly not patients. Be the physician who tells patients what they need to hear, not just what they think they want to hear (more on this in the section on Practicing the Art of Saying No in Chap. 12).

5.5.3 Use Your Influence When Warranted

Sometimes a test needs to happen urgently. You evaluate a patient with fatigue, weight loss, and jaundice. When you place the order for the right upper quadrant ultrasound, let the patient know that if it's not scheduled within a few days, you will advocate for an earlier appointment. If a test needs to happen right away, facilitate to make it happen.

I care for many patients who require heart transplantation. The evaluation process involves multiple blood tests, imaging studies, and consultations to confirm the patient's heart is sick enough while the rest of them is well enough to survive and thrive after transplant. Sometimes, the patient is ready to be listed save for a lagging consultant holding up the process. The patient may have a lung nodule on chest CT and the pulmonologist needs to see the patient, review the chest CT, and document their evaluation so the patient can either proceed to further expedited testing or transplant listing. Because having advanced heart failure warranting transplantation is the very definition of living on borrowed time, it is the cardiologist's responsibility to expedite the evaluation process so the patient can be listed as soon as possible. I had a mentor who would send good morning texts to lagging consultants at 7 AM, early enough to get their attention but not so early to as to be rude. These polite and cheerful reminders to consultants to evaluate scans and document findings met with terrific results and some consultants, over time, became more conscientious in their evaluations just to avoid the early-morning texts.

Patients may die while awaiting transplantation, and that is a tragedy. Patients may also die due to delays in the evaluation process and that is worse because it is preventable. This extreme situation is emblematic of all testing and interventions. Know when your influence is warranted to expedite testing and provide optimal patient care.

5.6 The Cases that Keep You Up at Night

As a junior physician I lived in fear of making the wrong decision, and there was another layer of dread: if something bad happened to a patient, would it have happened if a wiser and more experienced physician had been caring for the patient? The best antidote to this fear is to talk over the cases that keep you up at night with a trusted colleague/mentor.

Over the years, from many of these conversations, I gleaned what has become, for me, a reassuring mantra in the care of complicated patients: when you have done an appropriate and comprehensive assessment of the patient's symptoms and still cannot ascertain the diagnosis, give yourself permission to make peace with the lack of answers.

When you arrive at this place of acceptance, sharing your findings with the patient involves a combination of validation, tempered reassurance, and a plan with managed expectations.

5.6.1 Validation

It's important to emphasize to patients the difference between a negative test result and a lack of symptoms. Just because a stress test is normal doesn't mean the patient doesn't have chest pain. Just because the ambulatory ECG monitor doesn't show arrhythmias doesn't mean the patient doesn't have palpitations. If you focus on the normal test result instead of the symptoms, you are not fulfilling your responsibility to provide optimal patient care. The conversation doesn't end with a normal test result. A normal result does not mean your job is done.

5.6.2 Tempered Reassurance

I like to frame normal test results like this: "The good news is, the test is normal and we can exclude serious and dangerous causes like _____. The bad news is, we still don't know what's causing your symptoms so further investigation is needed to figure out how to help you feel better."

I cared for patient with fatigue and a low-normal ejection fraction on echocardiogram. Extensive evaluation for infiltrative heart disease even including cardiac

MRI failed to uncover a diagnosis and though the patient had fatigue, his exercise tolerance on stress test was normal.

I felt his fatigue was out of proportion to his cardiac findings, and that his low-normal ejection fraction was nonspecific. I didn't tell him he would be fine forever; short of a clairvoyant, who can provide such a guarantee? It was possible that he was in the early stages of a nonischemic cardiomyopathy. Still, as there were no lifestyle or medical interventions to halt potential progression, the most important management plan was to return to a generally healthy lifestyle with no restrictions.

5.6.3 A Plan with Managed Expectations

After tempered reassurance, the next step is to map out a plan to establish a diagnosis, which may involve the assistance of other specialists. When I explained to this patient that his low-normal ejection fraction was not the source of his fatigue and that conditioning from increased exercise might improve his symptoms, he was reassured. Just knowing that serious conditions have been ruled out may be enough to provide peace of mind and make the symptoms bearable. With this peace of mind, patients can move on to a plan of further evaluation or an acceptance of life with the symptoms.

Prepare the patient for the possibility that no diagnosis will be found despite further evaluation. The patient may have to learn to live with the symptoms. Finally, offer warning signs that could indicate a progression to a more serious diagnosis that would warrant more investigation.

5.7 The Worst-Case Scenario

What if the worst happens: your thorough evaluation yields no diagnoses and at some point in the future, the diagnosis is revealed, perhaps through repeating tests you already ordered or else a new test you had not initially considered? If the worst happens, you must dissect the case to understand if you went wrong, and how.

I saw a patient with incisional chest pain early after heart transplantation. I offered reassurance and pain medications. Three months after transplantation, the pain would not go away, which is unusual. I did not think he was inappropriately seeking narcotic pain medications, ' so by 4 months post transplantation, I referred him to surgery to assess if removal of sternal wires might help, as rarely, sternal wire removal alleviates prolonged incisional pain.

Imagine my shock when the preoperative CT scan showed sternal malunion, fragmentation, and surrounding soft tissue thickening raising the possibility of osteomyelitis. Imagine my greater shock tinged with horror when, intraoperatively, a sternal abscess was discovered. He ultimately required 2 surgeries for sternal debridement and reconstruction and a prolonged course of antifungal therapy for *Candida* osteomyelitis. After recovering from the second surgery and completing a course of antifungal therapy, he was a different person: his wan coloring was replaced with a healthy glow, he had more energy, and he looked happy for the first time since the transplant.

What was the lesson here? Should I have not minimized his pain and investigated his symptoms sooner? Fungal osteomyelitis of the sternum post heart transplantation is astonishingly rare, but should I have done a CT scan earlier in his course, instead of waiting to refer him to surgery 4 months after transplantation?

I got lucky: I referred him to surgery for the wrong reason and a subsequent CT scan uncovered the right diagnosis. I am relieved that he achieved a happy ending, that he bears no resentment, and that I learned an important lesson. When a patient has prolonged incisional pain after transplantation, don't assume it's because they have a low pain threshold; investigate the possibility of a sternal infection. That's the value of experience: this lesson has served me well in the care of subsequent patients.

You may never care for a post-transplant recipient with fungal osteomyelitis; there is a larger lesson here. If you're offering reassurance to a patient and you're not sure if reassurance is the right approach, talk to a trusted colleague or mentor. When a test uncovers a serious diagnosis that you didn't consider, seek out your mentors then too. Maybe you missed the diagnosis the first time, and if so, figure out why.

Was it because you, like me, didn't consider the condition on your differential diagnosis and thus didn't order the right test? Or was it because you ordered the right test and didn't consider the test characteristics, like how a stress test is only negative if the patient reaches target heart rate, and assumed an inadequate test was a normal one? There are situations where a false-negative, in light of your high pre-test probability, is less likely than a true negative and further investigation is still warranted.

Or did you miss the diagnosis because the patient was so early in the course of their disease that the testing would not reveal the diagnosis? Maybe it wasn't your fault; maybe it was a fluke. I cared for a heart transplantation who developed weight loss and jaundice 2 months after transplantation. One month later, he passed away from aggressive pancreatic cancer. Did I miss a pre-transplant diagnosis of pancreatic cancer? Thankfully, no: a standard pre-transplant screening chest and abdominal CT scan 5 months before transplant which showed a normal pancreas. While this was bad luck, tragic luck, it was not an error in medical judgment or reasoning.

This is a crucial dissection, between fault and fluke, and you have to get it right (see Chap. 13 for more on this). This patient's terrible outcome was a fluke, and flukes should not alter future management; the response is not to check performing screening abdominal CT scans on patients immediately before transplantation to assess for the vanishingly rare possibility of aggressive pancreatic cancer not seen a few months earlier. As the old joke goes, "What's the difference between God and a doctor?" The answer: "God knows he's not a doctor." Physicians are neither clairvoyant nor omnipotent. When something awful happens, sometimes the correct response is not to shoulder the responsibility—it is to accept that some bad outcomes are beyond our control.

Remember the adage "Good judgment comes from experience, and experience from bad judgment." Focus on learning the right lessons from your bad judgment.

Figure out first if your judgment was bad before you change your future practice based on it. Not every bad outcome warrants a change in practice and this scrutiny is essential to ensure that you gain the right experience.

5.8   The Golden Rule

When I was a medical student, I regarded the cardiologist's job as a straightforward and simple algorithm: a normal stress test means you're fine and an abnormal stress test means you need a stent. After residency and cardiology fellowship, I realized the algorithm had many more branch points and opportunities for subtle decision-making, because any therapeutic intervention must achieve a high bar of the Golden Rule: don't do anything to a patient if it won't help them feel better and/or live longer. Therapeutic interventions follow the same rules as diagnostic testing, with a major caveat: interventions generally carry more risk, so the bar for benefit must be met. As for corollaries to consider in adhering to the Golden Rule, consider the creeps; contraindication creep and indication creep, to be exact.

5.8.1   Contraindication Creep

Some medications have amazing evidence of benefit: think beta-blockers in patients with heart failure with reduced ejection fraction, or statins in patients with coronary artery disease. These medications also have contraindications. Beta-blockers are contraindicated in patients with asthma or chronic bronchitis/emphysema who wheeze more when on beta-blockers. Statins are contraindicated in patients who develop acute liver injury while taking them.

When I was a resident, I admitted a patient to the hospital with an acute myocardial infarction. He underwent stenting of the left anterior descending artery. When I presented his case to the attending physician on rounds the next morning, he asked me why the patient was not on a statin. I explained that the patient had biopsy-proven alcoholic cirrhosis awaiting liver transplantation and therefore a statin was contraindicated. This was the wrong answer and an example of contraindication creep. Statins should be avoided only if the liver enzymes (AST or ALT) are 2–3 times the upper limit of normal. Fortunately for the patient, my attending physician quickly corrected my mistake and the patient only went a day without statin therapy.

It is wrong to deny the life-saving benefits of beta-blocker therapy to any patient who carries a diagnosis of asthma or chronic obstructive pulmonary disease, or statin therapy to any patient with cirrhosis. If you're withholding an essential medication with proven benefit for quality of life or survival, make sure you're holding it for the right reasons. When in doubt, look it up—one happy consequence of the internet is that the facts are only a few clicks away.

5.8.2 Indication Creep

There is a tendency to be swept away with the excitement of late-breaking clinical trials (and the attendant jargon) at scientific meetings and to then apply the results to every patient you subsequently see. That's not always the right approach. Consider transcatheter edge-to-edge mitral valve repair. The COAPT trial compared transcatheter mitral valve repair to medical therapy for secondary mitral regurgitation in patients with heart failure (Stone et al 2018). In COAPT, the transcatheter mitral valve repair improved survival, hospitalization, symptoms, and quality of life.

Based on the results of COAPT, should a patient in the intensive care unit with cardiogenic shock and severe mitral regurgitation be whisked off to the cardiac catheterization laboratory for the cutting-edge procedure? No one knows; this is a data-free zone. When one is applying the basic tenets of "feel better, live longer" to an intervention, one cannot guarantee that this patient will benefit.

In the case of transcatheter mitral valve repair, it is even more telling that another randomized trial of patients with symptomatic heart failure with reduced ejection fraction and severe mitral regurgitation, the MITRA-FR trial, demonstrated no benefit from the transcatheter mitral valve intervention (Obadia et al 2018). The difference? MITRA-FR enrolled patients with large left ventricles, lower ejection fraction, higher pulmonary artery pressures, and less severe mitral regurgitation.

The lesson here: look at the patient population enrolled in the clinical trial. MITRA-FR enrolled patients with more severe heart failure, perhaps too advanced to benefit from the mitral valve repair. The 2020 ACC/AHA Valvular Heart Disease Guidelines appropriately consider these findings of differential benefit based on patient stability in their recommendations: the transcatheter mitral valve repair is not recommended in patients with severely reduced ejection fraction, severely dilated left ventricle, or severe pulmonary hypertension (Otto et al 2021).

Just imagine if MITRA-FR were the only randomized trial of transcatheter mitral valve repair for patients with heart failure and reduced ejection fraction—a useful therapy might have been discarded because it was tested in the wrong population.

There are many other examples of situations where you should guard against indication creep. Ivabradine is indicated for patients with heart failure and reduced ejection fraction only if the patient's heart rate remains over 70 in normal sinus rhythm on maximum-tolerated beta-blocker dose—because the landmark clinical trial of ivabradine, SHIFT, only tested benefit in such patients (Swedberg et al 2012). Isosorbide dinitrate and hydralazine are indicated only in patients with heart failure and reduced ejection fraction who are self-described as African American on maximum-tolerated doses of guideline-directed medical therapy—because the landmark clinical trial, A-HeFT, only tested benefit in such patients (Taylor et al 2004).

How should you avoid indication creep? Ensure that your patient meets criteria for the medication or intervention based on the enrollment criteria of the relevant clinical trials, the recommendations of expert consensus guidelines, and/or the indications on the FDA package insert.

5.9 "How Can It Hurt?" is Rarely the Right Justification

The opposing argument: just because a randomized clinical trial did not show benefit, should we deny our patients potential life-saving benefit of therapeutic interventions, whether medications or invasive procedures? While there is a tendency to "just give it a try," any student of clinical trials knows the dangers of this approach.

The road to bad outcomes is paved with wishful thinking, plausible pathophysiology, and surrogate endpoints (more on this in Chap. 13 in regard to Covid 19). Ask anyone who ever administered flecainide to suppress premature ventricular contractions (PVCs) after myocardial infarction (Echt et al 1991), post-menopausal hormonal therapy to improve lipid profiles (Manson 2003), or thiazoladinediones to reduce hemoglobin A1c in patients with diabetes (Lipscombe 2007). Reducing the burden of PVCs, the level of low-density lipoprotein cholesterol, and hemoglobin A1c are noble goals, yet medications to effect these changes result in arrhythmic death, coronary heart disease, and heart failure.

5.9.1 Be a Humble Student of Clinical Trials

There are also therapies that no one considered useful but showed unanticipated benefit in clinical trials. Consider beta-blockers, once contraindicated for heart failure, and now standard of care after trial after trial demonstrated survival benefit. Or phosphodiesterase-5 inhibitors, initially investigated for use in angina and hypertension, with the unexpected boon of fixing erectile dysfunction, thus spawning infomercials of baby boomers absurdly soaking in outdoor bathtubs; images we can never unsee.

Consider the greatest triumph in heart failure in the last decade, the SGLT2 inhibitors. After the thiazolidinedione debacle of surrogate endpoints (rosiglitazone was FDA-approved to treat diabetes based only on an improvement in hemoglobin A1c, a surrogate endpoint, and post-marketing surveillance demonstrated an increase in the risk of heart failure) (Lipscombe 2007), the FDA required that all future diabetic drugs be studied in cardiovascular outcome trials to document safety. No one expected that the SGLT2 inhibitors, when prescribed to patients with diabetes and cardiovascular disease or cardiovascular risk, would reduce the risk of heart failure, but that led to the genius leap of testing the impact of SGLT2 inhibitors in patients with heart failure *without diabetes* and a new pillar of heart failure therapies was established (McMurray et al 2019; Packer 2020).

The lesson: stay humble and be a student of clinical trials. It is difficult, sometimes, to "do nothing," even when doing "nothing" is the best therapeutic intervention. Be courageous by following the next corollary.

5.9.2 When in Doubt, Return to the Golden Rule

As a fellow, I rotated on the cardiology consult service with a senior, experienced attending. He was extraordinary, not just because he knew the names of everyone in the hospital, from the chief operating officer to the cafeteria lunch lady, but because he always knew when tincture of time was the right approach. Over the course of a few weeks, we received many consults for patients with abnormal stress tests or elevated troponin. Early in the rotation, I proposed an attempt at coronary revascularization for every patient (following my naïve one-size-fits-all algorithm of how I imagined cardiologists make decisions).

As I was presenting my plan, he would ask me how the results and subsequent intervention would help the patient feel better and live longer. He walked me through various scenarios: was I sure the patient's symptoms were consistent with angina? If their discomfort was not exertional and occurred while lying flat after eating, would an angiogram to assess revascularization options help them feel better? Of course, the answer was no; the patient needed lifestyle modifications to prevent gastroesophageal reflux disease with a time-limited trial of a proton-pump inhibitor and plans for endoscopic investigation if conservative measure failed. This attending physician was a master historian; through him, I learned to ask the pointed questions that uncovered one patient's ritual of eating peppermint patties in bed which turned out to a highly effective trifecta (chocolate, peppermint, supine position) for triggering heartburn.

If the patient had convincing stable angina and the stress test did not show a high-risk finding of a large area of anterior ischemia, multiple areas of ischemia, or a fall in ejection fraction with stress, was revascularization essential to improve quality of life and survival, or would aspirin, statin, and blood-pressure control be an appropriate initial approach? He was right again: the first step in the management of chronic stable angina is to treat the atherosclerotic process with a statin and the anginal process with beta-blockers, calcium-channel blockers, and nitrates. Treating the disease, not the stenosis, makes sense pathophysiologically, has been borne out in clinical trials, and is recommended in guidelines.

With every patient, he taught me how to approach every clinical situation with the Golden Rule, and how to use pathophysiology, clinical trials, and guidelines to chart the right course for my patients.

5.9.3 Bandaids versus Cures

Whenever you offer an intervention to a patient, ask yourself if you're giving them a bandaid, or a cure. For example, when a patient presents with iron-deficiency anemia, and you prescribe iron, you are addressing the diagnosis—but incompletely. The diagnosis doesn't end with iron-deficiency.

You have to ask yourself why is the patient iron deficient? It is a lack of dietary intake or related to blood loss? And if the latter, is it from menses or gastrointestinal losses? Has the patient had surveillance screening colonoscopies as recommended? Is there occult blood on fecal testing? If you give the bandaid of iron without investigating the source to offer the definitive cure, you have done the patient a disservice.

I saw a patient who was in his mid-50s with complete heart block. He was referred to a cardiologist who placed a permanent pacemaker. The pacemaker appropriately addressed the diagnosis—but incompletely. Why would a man in his mid-50s have complete heart block? No one asked and a few months later, while ice skating with his family, he sustained a polymorphic VT arrest. He was successfully resuscitated, and finally underwent additional evaluation which uncovered the diagnosis that had been brewing all along: cardiac sarcoidosis.

While his story has a happy ending: he emerged from the cardiac arrest unscathed and his cardiac function ultimately normalized with immunosuppressive therapy, it is a cautionary tale. Don't rest just because you have solved the immediate problem: investigate the etiology, or ensure that you have exhausted all avenues before you shrug your shoulders and move on.

5.10   Final Thoughts

There are no perfect tests, but there are systems to ensure you will make the most of the tests to make the right diagnoses. Remember to perform a thought experiment before you order any test. If you don't know the plan for a positive, negative, or indeterminate result, you should not be ordering the test. Once you order the test, remember to prepare the patient by communicating the urgency. Finally, when all the tests come up normal, but the patient still feels terrible, focus on the patient and not the normal findings. Provide validation, tempered reassurance, and managed expectations. When the worst happens—you miss a diagnosis—figure out why because improving your medical reasoning will help you to provide optimal care to your future patients.

When it comes to interventions, ensure you are meeting the high bar of the Golden Rule: it must make a patient feel better and/or live longer. Watch out for pitfalls: be a humble student of clinical trials to ensure you are choosing the right intervention for the right patient. Make sure your interventions are not simply band-aids—delve deeper to search and find the cure.

References

Echt DS, Liebson PR, Mitchell LB, Peters RW, Obias-Manno D, Barker AH, Arensberg D, Baker A, Friedman L, Greene HL, Huther ML, Richardson DW. Mortality and morbidity in patients receiving encainide, flecainide, or placebo. N Engl J Med. 1991;324:781–88.

Lipscombe LL, Gomes T, Lévesque LE, Hux JE, Juurlink DN, Alter DA. Thiazolidinediones and cardiovascular outcomes in older patients with diabetes. JAMA. 2007;298:2634–43.

Manson JE, Hsia J, Johnson KC, Rossouw JE, Assaf AR, Lasser NL, Trevisan M, Black HR, Heckbert SR, Detrano R, Strickland OL, Wong ND, Crouse JR, Stein E, Cushman M. Estrogen plus progestin and the risk of coronary heart disease. N Engl J Med. 2003;349:523–34.

McMurray JJV, Solomon SD, Inzucchi SE, Køber L, Kosiborod MN, Martinez FA, Ponikowski P, Sabatine MS, Anand IS, Bělohlávek J, Böhm M, Chiang C-E, Chopra VK, de Boer RA, Desai AS, Diez M, Drozdz J, Dukát A, Ge J, Howlett JG, Katova T, Kitakaze M, Ljungman CEA, Merkely B, Nicolau JC, O'Meara E, Petrie MC, Vinh PN, Schou M, Tereshchenko S, Verma S, Held C, DeMets DL, Docherty KF, Jhund PS, Bengtsson O, Sjöstrand M, Langkilde A-M. Dapagliflozin in patients with heart failure and reduced ejection fraction. N Engl J Med. 2019;381:1995–2008.

Obadia J-F, Messika-Zeitoun D, Leurent G, Iung B, Bonnet G, Piriou N, Lefèvre T, Piot C, Rouleau F, Carrié D, Nejjari M, Ohlmann P, Leclercq F, Saint Etienne C, Teiger E, Leroux L, Karam N, Michel N, Gilard M, Donal E, Trochu J-N, Cormier B, Armoiry X, Boutitie F, Maucort-Boulch D, Barnel C, Samson G, Guerin P, Vahanian A, Mewton N. Percutaneous repair or medical treatment for secondary mitral regurgitation. N Engl J Med. 2018;379:2297–306.

Otto CM, Nishimura RA, Bonow RO, Carabello BA, Erwin JP, Gentile F, Jneid H, Krieger EV, Mack M, McLeod C, O'Gara PT, Rigolin VH, Sundt TM, Thompson A, Toly C. 2020 ACC/AHA guideline for the management of patients with valvular heart disease: a report of the american college of cardiology/american heart association joint committee on clinical practice guidelines. Circulation. 2021;143:e72–227.

Packer M, Anker SD, Butler J, Filippatos G, Pocock SJ, Carson P, Januzzi J, Verma S, Tsutsui H, Brueckmann M, Jamal W, Kimura K, Schnee J, Zeller C, Cotton D, Bocchi E, Böhm M, Choi D-J, Chopra V, Chuquiure E, Giannetti N, Janssens S, Zhang J, Gonzalez Juanatey JR, Kaul S, Brunner-La Rocca H-P, Merkely B, Nicholls SJ, Perrone S, Pina I, Ponikowski P, Sattar N, Senni M, Seronde M-F, Spinar J, Squire I, Taddei S, Wanner C, Zannad F. Cardiovascular and renal outcomes with empagliflozin in heart failure. N Engl J Med. 2020;383:1413–24.

Stone GW, Lindenfeld J, Abraham WT, Kar S, Lim DS, Mishell JM, Whisenant B, Grayburn PA, Rinaldi M, Kapadia SR, Rajagopal V, Sarembock IJ, Brieke A, Marx SO, Cohen DJ, Weissman NJ, Mack MJ. Transcatheter mitral-valve repair in patients with heart failure. N Engl J Med. 2018;379:2307–18.

Swedberg K, Komajda M, Bohm M, Borer JS, Ford I, Dubost-Brama A, Lerebours G, Tavazzi L, Investigators S. Ivabradine and outcomes in chronic heart failure (SHIFT): a randomised placebo-controlled study. Lancet. 2010;376:875–85.

Taylor AL, Ziesche S, Yancy C, Carson P, D'Agostino R, Ferdinand K, Taylor M, Adams K, Sabolinski M, Worcel M, Cohn JN. Combination of isosorbide dinitrate and hydralazine in blacks with heart failure. N Engl J Med. 2004;351:2049–57.

Chapter 6
The Art of the Consult

I received the one and only rebuke of my medical career as a first-year cardiology fellow. I didn't mind spending all night on call in the hospital as a resident. I was single so rarely had any better place to be. I enjoyed the company of my co-residents: watching television with my colleagues in the residents' lounge after the admissions were tucked away for the night felt as much a social gathering as it did work. Those days, I had the enviable metabolism of a 20-something, so the cafeteria's breakfast-at-night menu of chocolate chip pancakes and Denver omelets was always a delight. Were there middle-of-the-night emergencies, unstable admissions, cardiac arrests? Of course, though the support of my on-call colleagues made even these difficult situations manageable. Together, we would brainstorm and stabilize sick patients. Camaraderie from my smart, kind, and funny colleagues, late-night television, and salty-versus-sweet breakfast-for-dinner dilemmas are what I remember most from call nights as a resident.

Call in fellowship was different and initially, I didn't handle it well. I was married and had responsibilities at home. Taking call from home added another dimension: the activation energy to rouse myself from bed to drive to the hospital was higher. Finally, my burgeoning ego borne of a little experience (though not enough) made me approach each call as an annoyance rather than an opportunity to help. I had just enough experience to be dangerous though my irritation was also a shield for my fear. There was also more pressure; as a fellow taking home call in the middle of the night, there was no coterie of supportive co-residents with whom to commiserate. Often, as I fumbled, bleary-eyed, through a stat echocardiogram, the cardiothoracic surgery fellow waited impatiently in the wings, ready to whisk the patient to the operating room based on my say-so.

As a fellow, I was balanced on the edge of experience. I was a full-fledged, board-certified internist, yet I had to again climb the steep learning curve, this time of a cardiologist. I had more authority and also more fear. The urgent consults in the middle of the night were more like real life and less like summer camp: would I get it right? The consults that were not so urgent also sparked annoyance, which is what led to my rebuke.

M. Kittleson, *Mastering the Art of Patient Care*,
https://doi.org/10.1007/978-3-031-20920-8_6

I was called in late one night to the surgical intensive care unit to see a patient with bradycardia. This was the days before smart phones, so the surgical resident who summoned me to the bedside in the middle of the night couldn't have just texted me a picture of the bedside monitor. If he had, I could have texted back a snarky education in taking a pulse and pointed out that the patient's heart rate was not 35, but 70, as the monitor was confused by ventricular bigeminy. The patient was also hemodynamically stable, adding insult to the injury of an urgent consult.

I raced into the SICU making no secret of my irritation. When the attending surgeon, also at the bedside, thanked me for my time, I did not respond graciously. When he told me he could do without my attitude, I replied that I could do without the consult (I cringe at the memory; it was not my finest moment). It turns out that surgeon had cared for a family member of the cardiology fellowship program director, and my program director called me to his office the next day.

Remarkably, my program director was kind. He did not lecture me on the importance of collegiality and professionalism. He seemed to realize that my rudeness was a result of fatigue and fear, not innate disrespect. He explained that while call was frustrating, when we were called to help, we had to be kind. At that moment, as he was gently chastising me, he provided a mentor moment, a terrific example on how to provide feedback tailored to the individual that starts with understanding rather than censure. He defused any defensiveness I might have had. Rather, I felt embarrassed because he was so kind.

Why am I telling you this story? So that you too will learn from your mistakes. This mistake hurt, and that was okay because embracing and learning from mistakes is important. Abdication equals inexperience. Learning from your mistakes is a rite of passage to experience. Consults are an art—both in giving and receiving—and here is my system for being the most effective giver and receiver of consults.

6.1 How to Call a Consult

6.1.1 Call Early

Consultants are not sitting around waiting for your call. When you are rounding on an inpatient and the team decides a consult is needed, call early. In the era of smartphones and electronic medical records, this can be accomplished efficiently while rounding. Consultants often spend part of the day in the hospital and part of the day in the office, fitting consults into an otherwise full schedule. The earlier you call the consultant, the sooner they can adjust their schedule to see the patient and provide recommendations in a timely fashion.

6.1.2   Have a Specific Question

A consultant's greatest annoyance is "I just want to have you on board." No one knows exactly what that means, except an opportunity to clutter the inpatient chart with say-nothing notes. There are three general reasons to call a consultant: (1) you are unsure of the diagnosis; (2) you are unsure of the management; or (3) you'd like a procedure performed that you cannot do yourself. Having a specific question is essential for two reasons: (1) the more specific the question, the more the consultant can help; and (2) a specific question requires that you have already reviewed the diagnostic and management plan and thus learned about the patient's condition, which adds to your experience and thus improves your patient's care.

Consider being unsure of the diagnosis: a patient presents with anemia. There is no evidence of blood loss based on history, physical, and fecal occult blood testing. The reticulocyte count is low, and there is no evidence of iron, B12, or folate deficiency. You note that the patient also has leukopenia and thrombocytopenia and have reviewed the patient's medication list without identifying potential culprits. You wonder if a bone marrow biopsy is indicated in this setting. This is a great reason for a consult—you have evaluated the patient to the best of your abilities, consulted trusty UpToDate, and applied the algorithm of differential diagnosis and testing as far as you can. When it is time to consider a specialized procedure, it's time to call the consultant. And imagine their delight when you say, "The patient has anemia with a low reticulocyte count consistent with decreased production but with normal iron, B12, and folate and associated leukopenia and thrombocytopenia. I cannot identify medications that might have contributed to the process and would like a consult to determine if a bone marrow biopsy is warranted." Contrast that with their chagrin if you were to call and say, "The patient has anemia—please advise and thanks in advance!".

A corollary to the rule of always having a specific question is that it's okay not to have a question if you're honest about why you don't. Sometimes a patient is sick, and you don't know what's going on. You're not sure if their constellation of symptoms has an infectious, rheumatologic, or endocrine source. In that case, be honest. Your uncertainty should not be a source of fear or worry. Concrete action plans are the antidote to fear and worry. Even if you cannot articulate exactly what help you need, facing uncertainty with a plan replaces stress with confidence. It's more than okay to call a consultant and ask for help: "I'm requesting a rheumatology consult because I am at a loss to find a unifying diagnosis for the patient's symptoms. I'm not sure if there is a rheumatologic source, and I would appreciate your expertise."

6.1.3   Tell the Patient

Many patients have been my mentors; when they suffer through mistakes, I have learned to be better. I admitted a heart transplant patient to the hospital with a new infiltrate on chest X-ray. Chest CT showed a mass, and the pulmonologist recommended a biopsy. How did the patient learn she had a lung mass? She found out when she asked her nurse why her breakfast tray was late. Her nurse told her that she wasn't getting breakfast that morning because she was scheduled for a lung biopsy.

When I rounded on her later that morning and saw the expression on her husband's face, after he raced to the hospital on the heels of his wife's frantic call, I was ashamed that the chain of communication had broken down so completely. Every physician caring for her, from the intern to the resident to the fellow to me, the attending physician, could recite the differential diagnosis for the lung mass yet none of us had explained the plan to the patient and her husband. Medical knowledge is critical for saving lives but almost meaningless without patient communication. Medical knowledge is taught; the art and importance of patient communication needs to be taught as well.

Does this seem like a minor point? It shouldn't. It happens all the time. Imagine being admitted to the hospital with a cough and finding out you have a lung mass from the nurse because you didn't receive the breakfast tray you ordered. Or, discovering that the biopsy showed cancer when an oncologist arrives, unannounced at your bedside, to discuss treatment options. Receiving bad news is bad enough (see section on Breaking Bad News in Chap. 9). Being blindsided by bad news is worse.

In the vein of "you break it, you buy it," if you order a test or a consult, take responsibility. Explain the results and the plan to the patient because you have a relationship with the patient. Before the patient is transported to the interventional radiology suite for a lung biopsy or oncologist arrives to discuss chemotherapy, explain the test results and prepare them for specialist consultations.

You must also make sure the patient agrees to the consultation; this is especially important for psychiatry consults. How I like to phrase it: "You seem depressed, which is understandable given all you are going through. Some patients benefit from seeing a psychiatrist who can offer coping strategies. Would you find this helpful?" Some patients say no; they do not believe psychiatrist can help them. Others are grateful for the opportunity. Either way, it's better for the patient, and the consultant, if you have explained the reason for the consultation before the consultant walks in the room.

6.1.4   Calibrate Your Concern

Being told that specialist consultation is required is nerve-wracking for the patient. As the physician, you might know that some consults will involve mainly reassurance. There is little urgency in a cardiology consultation for a newly recognized left bundle branch block in an asymptomatic patient. There is great urgency in a heart transplant consultation for a patient with multiple hospital admissions for decompensated heart failure. The patient may not know the difference. An otherwise healthy patient who's told that they have an "abnormal ECG" will assume the worst about their heart health.

When you advise an outpatient that they require a consultation, and you know that consultation is not urgent, let the patient know. In this situation: "I'd like you to see a cardiologist because your ECG is not completely normal. Because you have no symptoms, it's unlikely to be anything serious, though let's have a cardiologist weigh in to be sure. Continue all your usual activities and see the cardiologist within the next month. If the cardiologist's office can't fit you in, let me know, but a sooner appointment is not necessary." Provide the appropriate sense of urgency. Calibrate your concern so the patient can calibrate theirs.

In contrast, when a consultation is urgent, you must advocate on the patient's behalf to expedite the appointment. For example: "I am concerned that you have been admitted to the hospital with heart failure 3 times in the past 6 months and you need to see a heart failure specialist within the next 2 weeks. My office will expedite scheduling; I will call the specialist myself if needed." Again, you are calibrating risk and offering a concrete action plan.

There are moments when I have advocated directly on behalf of a patient for an urgent consult and I've never regretted it. There was a heart transplant patient that I had known for a decade who presented to clinic for a routine follow-up. As soon as I entered the examination room, I knew something was terribly wrong: her left arm and left leg were jerking uncontrollably with choreiform movements; she could barely maintain her balance on the examination table even with her daughter at her side to stabilize her. She told me the symptoms had been going on for 2 months after she was hospitalized with pneumonia and diabetic ketoacidosis and a local neurologist prescribed a benzodiazepine for anxiety.

This story made no sense. I had known this woman when she was dying of heart failure and in the early rocky months of recovery from heart transplantation and throughout all that, she was cheerful stoicism personified. Even I knew, as a cardiologist, that there was no link between choreiform movements and anxiety. I knew it could take weeks to get her an appointment with a neurologist. I couldn't bear to have her suffer a moment longer. I felt terrible that she thought anxiety was the problem when her anxiety was just the understandable by-product of the scary choreiform movements. And her suffering was significant: this formerly independent woman had taken leave from her work, was unable to drive or leave the house by herself, and her adult children were forced to put their jobs on hold to take turns caring for her.

I could not let her live another 2 months, suffering without answers, especially because I wasn't sure if she had a serious progressive neurologic disease that could benefit from immediate intervention. I considered sending her to the emergency room, but in the depths of the Covid pandemic, I didn't want to subject an immuno-suppressed patient to hospitalization. I was at a loss until I realized that there was a neurology clinic across the hall from the transplant clinic.

It was a one-in-a-million shot, but I dashed over to see if someone could help me. As luck would have it, one of the neurologists who specialized in movement disorders was in clinic that morning. I waited impatiently for him to exit an exam room and pled my case, even demonstrating her choreiform movements. He understood the urgency of her debilitating symptoms and saw her later that morning. After a thorough evaluation, he diagnosed her with hemichorea from diabetes, and I was relieved that she was finally in capable hands.

Did my clinic run a little late that day? Yes. Were patients upset? Not really, when I explained in general terms about the necessity of emergency consultation with a specialist across the hall. I emphasized how lucky my other patients were to not require emergency consultation. The look of relief on the patient's face, and her daughter's, when I returned to clinic to inform them that the neurologist was waiting to see them made it all worthwhile.

Communicating the appropriate sense of urgency applies to the consultant as well as the patient. Telling a consultant that a consult is urgent when it's not undermines your credibility and causes undue stress. Every physician has colleagues who request their patients be seen immediately when a delay of a day, for an inpatient, or a few weeks, for an outpatient, is medically appropriate. Providing a false sense of urgency indicates a lack of respect for the consultant. A false sense of urgency also clogs the system, diverting the consultant's time and energy away from truly urgent cases that require their experience. Don't be the referring physician who inappropriately fills the consultant's schedule with unnecessarily urgent consults. If you do this, it may be your next patient who truly needs an urgent consult and for whom there are no available slots. Don't be the boy who cried wolf.

You might argue that communicating this sense of urgency is part of advocating on the patient's behalf. Even if a consult is not medically urgent, you know the patient will worry about the issue until they see the consultant, so why not push the consultant to see the patient as soon as possible? Consider the patient described above with the abnormal ECG. What if the appropriate urgency is not explained to the patient, and they call the cardiologist, frantic, requesting an urgent appointment? The cardiologist might review the medical records and realize it's not at all urgent. The patient, on hearing this from the cardiologist's office staff, will be angry in addition to frantic, compounding one unnecessary emotion with another. Relaying a false sense of urgency to the patient makes life difficult for the consultant and, more importantly, causes unnecessary anxiety for the patient. As in all situations of life in general and medicine in particular, honesty and humility will serve you well.

This needless anxiety is also sometimes worse than a true medical urgency because it's very difficult to backtrack. Even if the cardiologist or referring physician attempts to reassure the patient that there is no medical reason for an expedited appointment, there will be a lingering sense of doubt, that the physicians are prioritizing convenience over their care. Prevent the unwarranted anxiety up front by being honest about the urgency of a consult and realistic about the timeline. Preventing unnecessary anxiety is better than attempting to assuage it.

Of course, sometimes you don't know whether a consult is urgent or not. If so—ask! There's nothing better than a consultant calling for advice on timing of the consultation. One of my patients showed up to her gynecologist's office to discuss fibroid surgery and her heart rate was 120 bpm. The gynecologist checked an ECG (insert bonus points here) which showed atrial fibrillation. The gynecologist could have sent the patient to the emergency department. Instead, the gynecologist observed that the patient looked and felt well and called me instead.

Since the patient carried a known diagnosis of atrial fibrillation, had no symptoms, and happened to miss a few doses of beta-blocker in the days prior, I was able to substitute close follow-up with me for an ED visit. This is a win–win: the patient was saved the hassle and expense of an unnecessary visit to the ED, the gynecologist was satisfied that she provided the best care, and the patient was reassured because her physicians were effectively communicating with each other and with her.

Might there be some consultants who are difficult to reach or unhelpful by phone? Of course. However, with time and experience, you will identify the consultants who are the most willing to help and these will form your go-to slate of experienced experts to turn to with difficult clinical dilemmas. What if you are new and inexperienced? You can always ask a trusted mentor or colleague for advice: which specialists do they rely on to provide optimal patient care?

6.1.5 Save the Plan for the Consultant

If a patient has chest pain and you order a stress test and the stress test is not normal, you will refer the patient to a cardiologist. While you should communicate the appropriate urgency to the patient, you should not communicate the plan. Not every stress test needs an angiogram. If the patient arrives at the cardiologist's office asking to schedule an angiogram, it's that much harder for the cardiologist to unring the bell of inappropriate information.

Maybe the patient's chest pain is not consistent with a cardiac source and the stress test findings are consistent with a false-positive artifact. Maybe the patient has chronic stable angina and a low-risk finding on stress test so optimization of medications is indicated prior to scheduling an angiogram. Whatever the subtlety, you are referring the patient to the consultant for their expert advice, so let them provide it.

This is what I would say: "Your stress test is not normal. This could be a sign of a blockage in a heart artery, and I'd like you to see a cardiologist to figure out the best plan. Sometimes medication adjustments are adequate and other times, a stent is needed. The cardiologist will let you know what approach is best for you." Offering the spectrum of potential interventions makes the consultant's job much easier: a clean slate to offer appropriate medical advice. It also makes your job easier; if you provide the consultant's plan to the patient before they see the consultant, and the plan differs, the consultant is not the only one who loses credibility: you do too.

Of course, I didn't realize this until I gained experience from my own mistakes. I saw a patient with symptomatic atrial fibrillation despite attempts at rate and rhythm control. I told her to see an electrophysiologist because she needed an ablation. However, the electrophysiologist felt that given her age and clinical history, ablation was unlikely to be successful. She lost faith in the electrophysiologist because she felt he was withholding important therapy and lost faith in me, believing that I send her to a substandard specialist.

It took a lot of explanation on my part, and a second opinion consultation, before she recognized the wisdom of not proceeding with an ablation. Now, when I refer a patient with symptomatic atrial fibrillation refractory to my attempts at rate and rhythm control, I'm careful to say that ablation is only one possible option and that I will defer the management plan to the expert. Sometimes the plan is an ablation and sometimes it's not; either way, the patient not only receives the best care, but trusts that they have.

6.1.6 Make Your Consultant Work for Your Patient

There are many ways to be an effective consultant, outlined later in this chapter. There are also ways to bring out the best in your consultant. A gastroenterologist once told me that whenever I was rounding on the inpatient heart transplant service, he always had to work a little harder. I took that as a compliment. He had to schedule urgent colonoscopies necessary for expedited heart transplant evaluations within a day and ensure his notes were accurate and internally consistent; if not, he'd have daily texts from me regarding schedules and clarifications.

If a consultant's note says the same thing every day while the patient's situation has changed, if the note doesn't offer contingencies for best/worst case scenarios, or if the plan outlined doesn't make sense or answer the question: reach out and ask! You have called a consultant for their expertise and if you feel unmoored by advice that is generic, contradictory, or incomplete, it is your duty to request clarification.

I cared for a patient awaiting heart transplantation who developed ischemic bowel and required small bowel resection and ostomy. The most important question, to my mind, was when the patient would be stable for re activation on the heart transplant waiting list. Yet every day, the surgeon's note focused only on initiation of tube feedings and wound care, so I reached out regarding the big picture. I asked for the specific surgical criteria required before the patient could withstand cardiopulmonary bypass and high-dose corticosteroid immunosuppression. The surgeon was helpful and future notes were tailored and relevant to this patient. Would it have been nice for the surgeon to intuit the relevant issues? Yes. Is it your job as the primary physician to guide and focus your consultants to answer the relevant questions? Also yes.

6.1.7 Know When to Push

Sometimes patients become my mentors when they suffer through mistakes, and I learn to be better. Other times, patients are mentors when I make the right choices and I'm empowered to apply the same successful lessons to the next patient.

A patient was referred to me for heart transplant evaluation. He had hemophilia and his local transplant center had declined him for prohibitive surgical risk. After reviewing his records, my first call was to an experienced hematologist who said that the patient would not be a candidate for transplantation at our center. Why? Because the laboratory would have to run Factor VIII activity levels every 2 h during the transplant operation and the hospital laboratory was not equipped to do this. The hospital lab only performed the test during business hours and transplant surgery could happen, without warning, at any hour of the day or night.

I could not accept that the barrier to transplantation was administrative and not medical. I asked her why the laboratory didn't perform the lab test 24–7. Answering this question required multiple meetings with lab directors and the heart transplant program's executive leadership. The end result: the necessary staff and training was arranged and the patient received his life-saving transplant.

The lesson here? Don't take no for an answer until you've exhausted all options. Use your consultants' experience and don't be afraid to push them in your attempts to distinguish real from perceived roadblocks to optimal patient care.

6.2 How to Be a Consultant

6.2.1 Be Prepared

When I receive a request for consult, whether inpatient or outpatient, I review the records in advance. For outpatients, this can result in more efficient care. There are times when I have diagnosed cardiac amyloidosis just on review of outpatient records and then arranged for the technetium pyrophosphate scan and monoclonal protein screen in advance, saving the patient multiple trips to the medical center and allowing more rapid diagnosis than if I had waited to review records on the day of consultation. I'm not just tooting my own horn: cardiac amyloidosis is in my sphere of expertise; don't expect me to diagnose interstitial lung disease or glomerulonephritis on the fly. Whatever your specialty, reviewing records in advance allows you to determine if there are gaps in the evaluation that you can fill on the day of consultation or prior, rather than waiting until afterwards.

With complicated patients, it's also helpful to gather the past medical history from the medical records, as opposed to from the patient's recollection. Whether they underwent an ablation for atrial fibrillation or re-entrant tachycardia, whether they have an implantable defibrillator with or without cardiac resynchronization therapy, or whether their prior intolerance to statin therapy included elevation in liver enzymes or just myalgias: establish these facts on chart review. Teasing out technical information from patients is not useful; rather, figure out how they feel. Whether the atrial fibrillation ablation or CRT-D implantation improved their symptoms, whether their muscle aches from rosuvastatin limited their activities: these are valuable points to confirm with the patient. Whether their QRS duration was above or below 150 ms at the time of CRT-D; for that, the medical records are key.

An additional bonus: preparation inspires confidence which in turn builds trust. If you are prepared, the patient knows that you are meticulous, detail-oriented, conscientious, and care about them. Patients who have confidence in you will trust you. Patients who trust you will be honest and open. Openness and honesty allow you to provide optimal patient care.

For inpatients, there are also advantages. As a specialist in heart failure and transplantation, I'm often asked to consult on inpatients in cardiogenic shock who may warrant urgent heart transplantation. It's no easy thing, to walk into a stranger's room and establish immediate rapport so that, in the space of a few minutes, they trust my recommendations regarding the life-and-death option of heart transplantation. You can earn this trust by being prepared. Comb through the chart and know everything about the patient before you enter the room. The more you know about them, the more they will confide in you. Preparation is one of the keys to uncovering the truth.

Know the indications for transplantation, the potential contraindications to transplantation, and have a plan to determine the right course for the patient. While your plan may change once you talk to and examine the patient, having a rough plan focuses you. Instead of becoming distracted by reviewing the chart as they speak to you, you can devote your full attention to their symptoms, goals, values, and preferences.

Consider a patient who traveled from another state for an outpatient heart transplant evaluation. She had been declined for transplantation and had received mixed messages about her candidacy along the way, which resulted in dissatisfaction and mistrust in addition to the disappointment of not being a viable transplant candidate.

I had painstakingly reviewed her records in advance because she had a complex surgical history as well as antibody sensitization; other transplant centers felt her surgical and immunological risk were prohibitive and deemed her ineligible. One note indicated that she had a 7-year-old son named (let's just say) Sean. When I walked into the examination room and saw her, her husband, and a little boy, I said, "You must be Mr. and Mrs. _____, and this must be Sean!" I could feel everyone in the room relax, Sean's smile the widest of all, because they realized that I cared, not just about her as a collection of diagnoses, but as a person. An unanticipated boon of preparation: knowing the details that make your patient a person.

When a patient realizes that you are prepared and they have your full attention, they are more likely to trust you. When I round on service with the internal medicine residents, they joke that I know the patients better than they do. They say, "You can't out-Kittleson Kittleson." I take that as a compliment and have the same goal with patients as I do with trainees: know your patient's medical history better than they know it themselves.

Preparation thus offers many advantages: (1) you save time in the gathering of facts; (2) you more efficiently formulate a diagnostic or treatment plan; (3) you effectively establish trust; and (4) you glean additional insight and information.

I have a few favorite lines that I share with patients at the start of a consultation, to establish trust and rapport. "I've had a chance to review your records, so I won't make you repeat a hundred things you've probably explained a hundred times. Let me refer to my notes and we'll get started." I also like, for patients with more complex medical conditions: "You may not know me, but I know all about you. It may be creepy when your neighbor says that, but it's comforting coming from a doctor, right? I've reviewed your chart in detail. I have a few questions and then we'll discuss the plan."

6.2.2 Be Specific

I have a catalog of cringe-worthy chart phrases that will be familiar to anyone who's ever read a consultant's note (see Chap. 2, Cringe-Worthy Phrases, for more detail—here you'll find the consultant-specific take on what not to write). Phrases like "gentle diuresis," "avoid nephrotoxins," or "consider XYZ" have no place in a consultant's note. Your job as the consultant is to be specific. Here are some examples of how to do that:

Gentle diuresis → the patient appears euvolemic; switch to Lasix 40 po BID with a goal I = O.

Avoid nephrotoxins → the patient is on ___ which may be contributing to acute kidney injury; replace with ___.

Consider XYZ is a big one. Consultants should not ask the physician who consulted them to consider among diagnostic and therapeutic options. The physician who consulted them did so because they weren't sure of the best plan; it's the consultant's job to stratify and prioritize and outline the appropriate approach.

An ineffective cardiology consultant would tell the primary team to "consider an angiogram." A useful cardiology consultant would instead offer: "An angiogram may be considered based on the patient's classic history of angina, but it does not appear to be unstable by history and there is no elevation of myocardial markers of injury. Thus, risk stratification with a stress test first is appropriate."

If you, as the consultant, feel the need to write "consider," ask yourself, why? Are you unsure of the best course of action? And if so, why are you unsure and what information would you need to become sure? While it is perfectly reasonable to share your uncertainty and thought process with the primary team that process doesn't end with "consider." Rather, it begins with "consider" and ends with a decision. A patient without a concrete action plan is a patient whose life is at risk.

When you feel yourself about to write "consider" in a note, rephrase to an "if, then" statement. So "consider angiogram" becomes "if the patient's troponin continues to rise accompanied by ongoing chest discomfort or ECG changes, then angiogram would be indicated."

6.2.3 Be Timely

As the only saying goes, a physician's most prized qualities are availability, affability, and ability (in that order). Performing a consult in a timely fashion is essential. As noted above, it's important that the person calling the consult offer you, the consultant, and the patient realistic expectations of how quickly the consult needs to happen. When the medical urgency is established, you should perform the consult within the medically appropriate timeline.

Timeliness doesn't apply just to how soon you see the patient; it applies to the consistency with which your relay your recommendations. We are lucky to live in the era of cell phones which allow rapid and efficient communication between primary teams and consultants. When I was a resident, my colleagues and I knew exactly where all the phones in the cafeteria were. When our pages went off in the midst of our breakfast-for-dinner feast, we knew which phone was closest and could dash there and back before the butter on our hotcakes congealed or our omelets cooled.

How lucky that you don't need to rely on the location of phones in the hospital cafeteria for timely communication. Reach out by phone, text, or email (the latter 2 without protected health information based on the encryption system and policies of your medical center) to update the consultant; unless the issue is truly straightforward, don't just leave a note for the primary team or send a note to the referring physician and assume it will be read. The direct contact allows for an exchange of ideas that fosters optimal patient care.

6.2.4 Be Part of the Team

In the ever-growing specialization of medicine, it's common for a sick and compli-cated patient to have multiple consultants who play crucial roles in their care. While patients may need many doctors, they also need a single, clear, unified message. As the consultant, discuss your plan with the primary team and other relevant consul-tants before you share your perspective with the patient. Don't put the patient in the middle of a management controversy, trying to play operator or translator.

Yet another example of patient as mentor: early in my career, I cared for a man who presented to the hospital with chest pain; based on troponin elevation in the setting of a normal coronary angiogram and inflammation on cardiac MRI, he was diagnosed with myocarditis. The management of myocarditis relies more on expert judgment than clinical trials: the decision to perform an endomyocardial biopsy or to administer corticosteroids or intravenous immune globulin is subject to much debate, even among experts in the field.

This patient had two cardiology consultants, the coronary care unit cardiologist and me, the heart failure specialist. As the heart failure specialist, I felt an endomy-ocardial biopsy was warranted to exclude giant cell myocarditis. The cardiologist in the intensive care unit did not and told the family so before we had a chance to discuss the patient together.

This put me in a difficult position. Families don't need to be caught in the middle of medical disagreements so, before talking with the family, I approached the cardi-ologist. While he was not entirely convinced that an endomyocardial biopsy was indicated, he agreed to present a unified front to the family. He supported the deci-sion to proceed with a biopsy since the evidence and guidelines were not clear and I had greater experience managing myocarditis.

Our conversation to achieve consensus was especially helpful when I finally spoke to the patient and his family. They agreed to an endomyocardial biopsy which showed giant cell myocarditis. The patient received immunosuppressive therapy and he was lucky: he ultimately recovered and was discharged from the hospital.

When there is a difference in opinion between physicians, families should hear about the different perspectives. However, families should not be expected to make medical decisions. In this case, the family benefited from our consensus-building process. The lessons here: conversations are better than chart wars, and disagreements between physicians should be settled between the physicians and not mediated by patients.

6.2.5   Anticipate Questions

When I perform a consult, my goal is to provide enough information so that the primary team can adequately care for the patient. If the primary team is unsure of the plan based on my note and has to call me to clarify, I have failed. Precious time and energy that could be spent on patient care should not be wasted trying to track down the consultant.

As a consultant, how can you anticipate questions? Sometimes, it's because you performed a consultation for a similar issue before, and then received multiple calls with requests to clarify or extend your recommendations. Other times, it's because your attending physician, when reviewing the consult with you, asked you how you would handle contingencies related to the consult question. What if you haven't had the experience and don't have a mentor to guide you? Do the thought experiment considering related issues and address them. Don't forget to include recommended outpatient follow-up and at what interval if warranted. These strategies will help you cross the bridge from inexperience to experience and provide more useful consults.

For example, if I'm asked to assess a patient for a preoperative cardiac evaluation, I anticipate issues. I will note if the patient is at acceptable cardiac risk to proceed with surgery and provide guidance on how long antiplatelet and anticoagulant medications may be safely held. If the patient has paroxysmal atrial fibrillation, I'll add a sentence: "The patient will likely go into atrial fibrillation related to the stress of surgery, but as her ejection fraction is normal and she has no history of heart failure, she will tolerate this well and this can be managed with a temporary increase in rate control medications as needed." If the patient has hypertrophic cardiomyopathy, I'll add: "Due to left ventricular outflow tract obstruction, the patient will be sensitive to hypovolemia and may become hypotensive. This is best managed with intravenous fluids and vasopressors such as phenylephrine or vasopressin in refractory cases."

In addition to anticipating issues, I like to offer longer-term recommendations. For example, for a patient with atrial fibrillation with rapid ventricular response, if I recommend amiodarone, I'll provide the starting dose and recommendations for the taper: "Amiodarone 1 mg/min IV for 6 h followed by 0.5 mg/min for 18 h, then amiodarone 400 mg twice daily for 10 days and then 200 mg daily until outpatient follow-up."

While it's important to anticipate issues, it's also important to not overstep. When I was a medical student, I would write "consider cardiac anesthesia" in every consultation to assess preoperative cardiac risk because I had read that in other notes written by other inexperienced physicians. Of course, the "consider" was all wrong, as we've discussed. So was the "cardiac anesthesia" part.

I later rotated with an anesthesiologist whom I admired. He would spend the quiet hours of surgery quizzing me on pathophysiology. My first grilling on Ohm's Law and the circulatory system came from this anesthesiologist. He also provided his perspective on preoperative cardiovascular risk assessments. He explained what cardiac anesthesia entailed, how it was not always appropriate for every patient with prior cardiac disease, and how it would misdirect a relatively scarce resource away from patients who truly needed it. An inappropriate recommendation for cardiac anesthesia puts anesthesiologists in a bind, much like the referring physician who paints a consultant into a corner by telling the patient what diagnostic/therapeutic interventions are needed before they see the consultant.

I gained many lessons from this anesthesiologist during our two weeks together, from shock physiology to the importance of respecting a specialist's scope of expertise. I knew I was not going to become an anesthesiologist, yet this medical student rotation allowed me to appreciate the impact of one specialty on another. Now, when I provide a consultation, I try to view the practicality and relevance of my recommendations on other specialists when our fields overlap. Medicine is a team sport; respect the knowledge and experience of other team members. Do not overstep the boundaries of your specialization. Do unto other experts as you would have them do unto you.

Because of this fleeting mentor, I do not dictate specifics of intraoperative cardiac monitoring when I provide preoperative cardiovascular risk assessment. I will not say, "The patient should have anesthesia provided by a cardiac anesthesiologist with intraoperative monitoring with a pulmonary artery catheter and arterial line." I don't do this because I am not the expert in anesthesia; I am an expert in cardiology. What happens in the operative room is at the discretion of the anesthesiologist.

Instead, I may say, "The patient is at increased risk for surgery given a history of nonischemic cardiomyopathy but is at acceptable risk given the importance of the surgery and because he is well-compensated with no evidence of heart failure. However, he would be at increased risk for perioperative volume overload and hypotension, and I will defer to the anesthesiologist to decide if intraoperative monitoring with a pulmonary artery catheter and arterial line is indicated." Don't back other specialists into a corner with your recommendations; offer your expertise and let them exercise theirs.

6.2.6   Know When to Sign Off

One of the most unsatisfying parts of medicine is when you feel you are not helping a patient. If you are consulted on a patient, and the issue for which you have been consulted has resolved, then it's time to sign off. One way to know it's the right time to sign off: you're writing the same thing in the chart and saying the same thing to the patient day after day.

There is a right way and wrong way to sign off a consult. The wrong way is to silently disappear from the chart without warning. The right way is a 2-step process: (1) document the signoff in your note: "I will sign off as there are no acute cardiac issues. Please contact me at ___ if issues arise;" and (2) contact the referring physician directly and explain why you are signing off.

Signing off prevents confusion for the patient with multiple consultants, reduces chart clutter which impairs effective communication, minimizes medical waste through unnecessary billing, and allows you to focus on patients who require your expertise.

6.3 How to Work Together

6.3.1 Avoid Chart Wars

Sometimes, as a consultant, you offer recommendations, and they are not followed. Other times, you call a consult and do not follow the recommendations provided. There is a right way, and a wrong way, to handle these instances.

I cared for a patient with heart failure with reduced ejection fraction who was admitted after an inappropriate defibrillator shock for atrial fibrillation. An electrophysiologist recommended propafenone. Though I knew that propafenone was a Class IC antiarrhythmic not recommended for patients with reduced ejection fraction, I did not reach out to the consultant to discuss. Instead, I wrote a note in the chart indicating that propafenone was contraindicated and stopped the medication.

In my inexperience, I created a shortsighted and ultimately destructive chart war. The right course of action would have been to communicate directly with the consultant. If I had, I would have realized that the patient had documented intolerance to several other antiarrhythmic medications, had prior attempts at ablation, and was aware of the potential risk of propafenone.

As the consultant later explained when he reached out to me, propafenone was the next best step. Now, if he had documented his reasoning in the chart, perhaps I would not have resorted to a chart war (see *Anticipate issues* outlined earlier in the chapter). Nonetheless, when you disagree, reach out first and document later. I learned this lesson the hard way, but you don't have to. Use my bad judgment to inform your experience and do better.

The right answer is always to reach out directly. If you are not following the recommendations of your consultant, reach out, explain why, and consider the consultant's reasoning behind their recommendations. If the referring physician is not following your recommendations, reach out and explain your reasoning. Sometimes, there is a misunderstanding on the part of the referring physician, or the consultant and consensus can be achieved. Sometimes, the referring physician and the consultant will continue to disagree. In this situation, the consultant may choose to sign off or the referring physician may seek out another opinion. Either way, the patient has received optimal care because a direct discussion of complex issues has not been reduced to a chart war.

6.3.2 Pick Your Battles

Sometimes there is no right answer in a disagreement. I care for patients in the cardiothoracic surgical intensive care unit (CSICU) after heart transplantation. In the CSICU, intensivists, cardiac surgeons, and heart transplant cardiologists are all eagerly involved in the early post-transplant management, so I pick my battles wisely. I will take a firm stand on the indications for induction immunosuppression and titration of tacrolimus to achieve therapeutic levels. If the intensivist wants to prescribe furosemide 40 mg IV every 4 h when I think furosemide 80 mg every 12 h is enough, I will not intervene. If the surgeon wants to keep the patient on epinephrine and nitroglycerin infusions for the first 48 h after transplant and then add amlodipine for hypertension, I will inwardly wince at the inelegance of this regimen and keep my own counsel.

There is style, and there is substance. If the patient has progressive renal dysfunction due to inappropriately aggressive diuresis, or tachyarrhythmias from excessive adrenergic stimulation from vasoactive agents, I will make some noise. Otherwise, I choose wisely where to spend my currency of influence. I keep my daily recommendations focused on my immunosuppressive sphere of expertise. I stray into areas of post-surgical hemodynamic management only when I feel that more than my delicate sensibilities will be affected by inelegant medication choices. If you choose your battles wisely, you are more likely to be heard. When you choose wisely, people know that when you speak, it's important to listen.

6.4 Final Thoughts

Medicine is becoming more specialized every day. I remember sitting in the medical school library as a second-year student, despairing over the seemingly impossible-to -understand organization of interstitial lung diseases when 3 tomes on a nearby shelf caught my eye. The title of this 3-volume set? "Cornea." I realized that if the cornea, which didn't even have a blood supply, could take up that much space on the bookshelf, there was no hope of me knowing everything. That might have been a breaking point—but it wasn't. Realizing that I could not have all the answers meant that medicine would be a team sport—and you, too, will optimize patient care with multidisciplinary collaboration with your consultants.

Part III
Establishing Your Medical Style

Chapter 7
Good Habits for a Lifetime

So much of your style and personality as a physician is cemented in medical school. Because much of medicine is an apprenticeship, you will learn by observing and modeling yourself after those you admire. At times, it is just a fleeting moment that makes an enormous difference. I worked with an amazing ophthalmology resident on a 2-week rotation as a fourth-year medical student. Truth be told, I picked the rotation because I heard it would be easy and I had already matched in internal medicine. I did not expect to work with an eager resident who changed the way I cared for patients. His enthusiastic lessons on the phoropter to determine eyeglass prescriptions did not stick, but the way he examined patients has impacted my practice even now, decades later.

Whenever he auscultated a patient's heart or lungs, he would consciously put his hand on their shoulder too, leaning in. He explained that he wanted the patient to know that he was fully engaged and committed to the examination. He didn't want the patient to feel only the touch of the stethoscope because he thought they would assume that he only cared about them as a collection of organs instead of as a person.

To this day, eyeglass prescriptions remain as intelligible to me as Cyrillic characters. However, I have never forgotten his approach to the physical examination. Every time I examine a patient, I place my hand on their shoulder as I place my stethoscope over their chest or back. This small gesture does build connection and I think of him.

Valuable knowledge will come from sources that you least expect, like that grumpy cardiothoracic surgeon I met on my first rotation as a third-year medical student. He was not interested in teaching medical students in general or me in particular. Nonetheless, I caught a glimpse into the world of pediatric cardiothoracic surgery by paying attention to the discussion between him and his fellow as they dissected a walnut-sized heart and made plans for the infant's future. Keeping an open mind will allow you to absorb the styles and practices of many fleeting mentors who may inform your medical practice for a lifetime. Here are what I consider to be the most important tools to take with you from medical school to your future career as an outstanding physician.

M. Kittleson, *Mastering the Art of Patient Care*,
https://doi.org/10.1007/978-3-031-20920-8_7

7.1 Preparation

Interns pre-round. As an intern, I would fantasize about the luxurious life led by my senior residents and attendings. These giants in the field strolled into rounds, listened to my presentations, gave a few bits of advice, and sauntered off to have coffee. Of course, once I became a senior resident, and then an attending physician, I realized there was little strolling and sauntering to be done, because pre-rounding is not just for interns (an there is seldom any time for coffee).

Here are the most important components to the art of pre-rounding:

(1) Don't wake up the patient. Is there anything worse than creeping into a patient's room in the wee hours of the morning (that feel more like the dead of night), turning on the light (or leaving the light off and whispering at them in the dark), and inquiring about bowel movements or shortness of breath? Yes, there is something worse: making them sit up in bed so you can auscultate their lungs which will undoubtedly have bibasilar crackles due to atelectasis because they are not awake enough to take deep breaths. If the patient is awake, perform the subjective (S) and objective (O) of your SOAP note. If they are asleep, you may note on attending rounds that you chose not to interrupt their much-needed sleep and deferred the physical examination to attending rounds.

(2) Know what happened overnight. The best way to figure this out is to review orders and nursing notes. If it's not in the nursing note and nothing new was ordered, then it's a good bet that nothing exciting happened overnight.

(3) Know the results of any imaging studies and consult recommendations that weren't available at the end of the prior day. Electronic medical records have many downsides (as covered in Chap. 2). The greatest upside is the ability to quickly and efficiently biopsy the chart for this information.

This art of pre-rounding applies to interns, residents, fellows, and attending physicians alike. When I was an intern, my pre-rounding plan took up a page—per patient. As a resident and fellow, I summarized each patient on an index card. As an attending physician, I have one line for each patient and a few general checkboxes regarding the big picture.

I formulate this concrete action plan before I round with the residents and fellows for three important reasons: (1) you won't waste time on rounds confirming the accuracy of the trainees' presentation by reviewing the chart as they talk; instead, you can critique the quality of their presentations; (2) you can take the time to think through the issues and formulate best management strategy for the patient in advance; and (3) you can devote more time to teaching rather than looking up laboratory studies and consultation notes on rounds.

Learn to pre-round efficiently as an intern and then use this skill as an attending physician to optimize your teaching and patient care.

7.2 The Worst-Case-Scenario Game

Benjamin Disraeli said, "Hope for the best, prepare for the worst." This adage applies well to medicine. When I was a resident on call in the CCU, I used to play the worst-case-scenario game with my interns. At the end of the night, I would ask the intern what was the worst thing that could happen to each patient over the next 12 h and what was their plan for that possibility. This strategy forced interns to confront uncertainty and combat worry with a concrete action plan.

Continue this exercise throughout your career. If you have a nagging fear about a patient, ask yourself what you are most afraid of and what you should do if it happens. If you can't put a name to the fear, or if you can't figure out a plan for that worst-case scenario, then look it up and/or ask for help.

Which brings us to the next important habit-for-a-lifetime.

7.3 Don't Be Afraid of What You don't Know

You're never too important to ask for help. It's more important to know the right question than the right answer. Sometimes, help will come from UpToDate or a review article or a guideline document. Sometimes, it will come from a chat with a trusted colleague. Regardless, take the time and energy to figure out what you don't know. This directed learning is how you gain practical knowledge that will stick.

When you care for a patient with a given disease, the questions about management are more practical and relevant. In medical school, I dutifully memorized the pathophysiology, clinical manifestations, laboratory testing, and management of the cardiac sequelae of carcinoid syndrome. Still, it took a patient to place the memorization in a clinical context.

I knew theoretically that left-sided valvular disease could be encountered in up to one-third of patients with carcinoid syndrome in the presence of patent foramen ovale (PFO) with right-to-left shunt, bronchial carcinoid, or high circulating levels of vasoactive substances overwhelming the hepatic and pulmonary degradative capacity. These facts achieved useful relevance when I was faced with a patient with carcinoid syndrome. To counsel her on her risk for cardiac involvement, I had to confirm whether she had a PFO, lung involvement, or high levels of carcinoid factors. Dry paragraphs in a textbook are important to form the foundation of medical knowledge; patients (literally) bring the facts to life.

You'll also find that giving a talk on a given topic forces you to understand it. In crafting a talk, you will consider your audience and make slides to address anticipated questions and practical concerns. You will explain concepts clearly and look up the questions for which you don't have answers. For example, when the PARADIGM-HF trial was published in August 2014 (McMurray et al 2014), I was excited, but paid the subtleties little attention. I knew it was a landmark trial as it was the first time since 1987 that a medication, sacubitril/valsartan, was proven superior to an

ACE inhibitor in patients with heart failure with reduced ejection fraction. I was also pregnant and had a toddler running around—so meditation on the finer points of this brand-new class of medications could wait.

Fast-forward to the Fall of 2015, when I was asked to give a 10-min talk on sacubitril/valsartan, newly approved by the Food and Drug Administration. I was still overwhelmed (now with a toddler and an infant) though the looming talk deadline forced me to digest the subtleties of the trial.

I'm grateful for the motivation this talk provided. I delved deeper into the rationale for the combination of sacubitril, a neprilysin inhibitor, with valsartan, an angiotensin receptor blocker. I researched the past studies of neprilysin inhibitors and ACE inhibitors. I knew physicians would need to know the indications, contradindications, and alternatives so they would be empowered to prescribe the medication and able to explain why to their patients. The lesson: use whatever impetus available, whether a patient with an unusual condition or a looming talk deadline, to jumpstart your learning.

The worst way to learn is to read about a random disease in a textbook. A better way to learn is look up the answer to a specific question about the patient in the textbook. The very best way to learn is to teach what you've learned to someone else. When knowledge has context, its importance becomes clear and it's almost impossible to forget.

7.4 Checklists: Not just for Interns Anymore

A senior resident once told me that there were two kinds of interns, those who made checklists and those who put patients' lives in danger. Fastidious attention to detail saves lives. Conscientiousness never goes out of style, and there's nary a sight more heartwarming to an attending physician than an intern making checklists on rounds. Interns who make lists are interns who are building the foundation of optimal patient care.

Checklists aren't just for interns, though. Residents, fellows, and attending physicians must be reliable: devise a system that works for you. My system on the inpatient service is a printout of patient names with checkboxes of what I need to do every day. The tasks may include: call the referring physician with an update, harass the consultant who leaves incomplete recommendations (more on managing consultants in Chap. 6), discuss the inaccuracies in the note with the intern. My system on the outpatient service is a list I email to myself at the end of clinic: clarify the urgency of non-cardiac surgery in a patient with a recent stent, send a condolence card to the widow of a patient who has passed away.

Checklists keep you honest, humble, and reliable—important qualities to have over a lifetime in medicine.

7.5 Time Management

When I was a trainee shadowing an attending physician in her outpatient clinic, the nurse would pop in her office to let us know a patient was ready. I would jump up, ready to see the patient, as my attending physician kept chatting away, seemingly oblivious to the patient waiting in the exam room a few doors down. This bad example stayed with me; this attending physician was a role model of what not to do. Doctors should have an allergy to keeping people waiting or being late. Your patients' time is as valuable as yours—do your best to be on time. This strategy is also a win—win situation: after more than 15 years in practice, my patients are conditioned. They arrive early for their appointments and often tell me that they do so because they know that I'll see them on time. Don't be the doctor who runs late and makes the patients late: don't be the rate-limiting step in your schedule.

Now, some patients will be late themselves, or make you run late because they need more time and attention. You can build this buffer into your schedule if you prepare electronic charts in advance, so that the records of relevant history have been abstracted and majority of the plan is roughly anticipated/templated. In this manner, the bulk of the visit is not spent rehashing their medical history but focusing on current symptoms and the plan.

Preparing in advance also allows me to enjoy the respite from medical talk when patients want to spend a few minutes discussing their growing family—or mine. (An aside: allow the patient to initiate discussions about your personal life. If the patient asks first, still keep it short and sweet. They have come to you, along with the 20 other patients on your schedule, for help, not social hour.)

The other key to time management is to always be doing something. I worked with a physician whose efficiency was astonishing. She saw a high volume of patients, had administrative leadership responsibilities, and still left work every day in time to pick her kids up from school. What was her secret? She told me that 5 min earlier in the day was worth 30 min by the end of the day: in other words, any little pocket of time is an opportunity to get work done. Instead of spending these pockets of time chatting with colleagues by the watercooler, she would prep a few notes for clinic, read an echocardiogram, or complete a mandatory wellness webinar.

I appreciated the insight of this fleeting time-management mentor: lots of little work does not require an uninterrupted swath of time. Fill in the tiny free intervals in your day with the minor tasks, because 5–10 min of found time between patients adds up to 30 min of family time later in the day. The happy consequence of this approach: you will become an anti-procrastinator.

7.6 Be Nice and Work Hard

As the director of the advanced heart failure and transplant cardiology fellowship, I meet with the fellows for an orientation every June. I tell them the year will involve a lot of hard work and a lot of learning—and their hard work will be in the service of learning. We will protect them from scut (waiting by fax machines for culture reports from hospitals) in favor of service (spending hours at a patient's bedside titrating vasoactive agents while discussing the plan for temporary mechanical support with the patient, family, and cardiothoracic surgeon). I promise to protect them: if they feel disrespected or worse, it is my job to address the problem. Rather than entering fellowship armed with a fully-formed fund of knowledge, I ask them to be nice and work hard. How can you accomplish this? Consider the most important qualities to adopt as a trainee and encourage and instill in trainees are: (1) choose kindness and (2) be reliable and respectful.

New trainees are often very nervous. Do they know enough? Are they good enough? In fact, the least important priority for trainees is fund of knowledge; if a trainee knew everything already, what's the point of training? What really matters is attitude and initiative; be nice and work hard because attitude and initiative are more important than aptitude and fund of knowledge.

Be nice because the village required to properly care for complex patients requires a multidisciplinary team and it is essential to learn to work well as members of a team. This requires the ability to listen, take everyone's views into perspective, and to disagree civilly. Work hard because your patients' lives depend on it. Part of expecting integrity is to model integrity.

In *A Bronx Tale,* Sonny LoSpecchio was asked, "Is it better to be loved or feared?" He replied, "That's a good question. It's nice to be both, but it's very difficult. But if I had my choice, I would rather be feared. Fear lasts longer than love." This Machiavellian sentiment may play well in an American crime movie, but is not useful in the hospital. Fear is not the same as respect. Model kindness and aim to be respected but never feared.

7.6.1 Choose Kindness

On call, I would often answer pages with, "What's the emergency?" My words, and my tone, reeked of grudging forbearance: why should my sleep be interrupted for issues that I knew were routine? I knew that a blood pressure of 160/90 mm Hg at two in the morning was not an emergency; the only impact would be an elevation in my blood pressure in response to the call. Lacking empathy and experience, I failed to realize that a minor irritation to me might feel like an emergency to a patient.

Then, late one night, my toddler spiked a high fever. I spent an hour worrying whether I should call the pediatrician and another hour second-guessing whether I should just wait until morning. All the while, his temperature was rising. Finally, I decided to navigate the complicated middle-of-the-night answering service phone tree that culminated in a voicemail. I spent a fraught wait, ready to snatch the phone, mid-ring, so as not to wake the rest of the family when the pediatrician called back. By the time I had the pediatrician on the phone, my nerves were shot. Her first words were, "How can I help?".

In the middle of the night, so worried about my kid, I almost burst into tears. I was so relieved that she opened with kindness, not impatience. I was also ashamed that I could have made middle-of-the-night callers feel badly when they had reached out to me for help. This pediatrician became a fleeting mentor. Now, I answer every call with, "How can I help?" and it sets the most amazing tone for every call. Being rude will not limit calls or inspire trust, though it will make them less pleasant for all involved.

7.6.2   Reliability and Respect

When I was on the precipice of fellowship, about to emerge from the chrysalis of training, once and for all, for the real word of attending-hood, I received an astonishing piece of advice. One of the interventional cardiologists told me that the best way to make 100 monkeys behave was to kill just one. He had an unconventional style of practice with patients and trainees alike, and while it worked for him, I was unconvinced that ruling by fear would work for me. (And it certainly wouldn't work for that dead monkey.)

Instead, I decided that I would do my best to live by another attending's advice. He told me that I should strive to be known as a physician who is reliable and held in high esteem by the nursing staff, and for me this sums up the qualities one requires to take the best care not only of patients, but also of colleagues, as strong and respectful working relationships will enrich your life and the care you provide to your patients.

A cardiology attending once wrote only two words on my fellowship evaluation, "100% reliable." At first, I was stung. There were so many other things I wished he'd said: great fund of knowledge, strong clinical judgment, kind to patients. Then I realized that being reliable encompassed all that. A reliable physician is one that can be trusted both by members of the medical team to embrace the shared mission of optimal patient care, and by patients to save their lives.

We all know that certain attending physician who will never respond to text messages, phone calls, or emails. We have all been in the position of having to track them down in person and when we do, having to then pin them down for a specific and helpful response. We all know the moment of dread when we realize that we need that one particularly elusive physician because they are on call or the only physician capable of addressing the problem.

If I have a close relationship with such a physician, I will let them know their behavior frustrates me. One highly specialized consultant apologized and told me that every time I email him, I should text him to let him know that I've sent him an email because otherwise he forgets to check email. Now, it's not my job to instruct him on email etiquette and responsiveness, so I dutifully accompany each email with a text alert. He now responds immediately to urgent requests and together, we can provide optimal patient care. While this is a lesson in working around roadblocks and figuring out how to get the job done for your patients, your goal is to never be him. Instead, be the trusted and reliable source that others can count on.

How do you become a reliable physician? Timely communication is the most important step. Return phone calls within 24 h. Answer emails within 24 h, if only to say you have received the message and will respond with a definitive answer in X amount of time. Delegate administrative tasks to your nursing and administrative staff. Imagine in you were patient awaiting a test result and were told it would be available in 2−3 days. Four days pass, and no word, because someone (doctor, nurse, assistant) dropped the ball and neglected to call you. You would be distraught, and unnecessarily. Whenever I review test results, I try to empathize with the patient, worried and dangling, and do my best to always close the loop.

Reliability sums up so many important qualities of a good physician: you do what you say, you say what you do, you respond promptly, you are prepared. Being held in high esteem by the nursing staff means that you are not only reliable, but that you are respectful. You will admit fault, be honest when you don't know the right answer, and you will not be rude just because you can be rude−always stay humble.

7.7　Final Thoughts

What do all these attributes have in common? They are facets of conscientiousness, and in medicine, conscientiousness is an essential component of compassion. The more you strive to be reliable and prepared, the better care you will provide to your patients—and it is never too early (or too late!) to cement good habits for a lifetime in medicine. Your patients will benefit and you will experience the joy of optimal patient care.

Reference

McMurray JJ, Packer M, Desai AS, Gong J, Lefkowitz MP, Rizkala AR, Rouleau JL, Shi VC, Solomon SD, Swedberg K, Zile MR, Investigators P-H, Committees. Angiotensin-neprilysin inhibition versus enalapril in heart failure. N Engl J Med. 2014;371:993–1004.

Chapter 8
Leading Your Team

8.1 Tough Transitions: Being a Leader

Being an intern didn't worry me much. Just as the first two years of medical school were like an extension of the didactic college experience, intern year was an extension of the clinical rotations of medical school. While internship involved more patients and longer hours, a safety net of residents, fellows, and attendings would always be there to break my fall. Interns are responsible only for themselves and never make a decision without someone more senior looking over their shoulder and nodding encouragingly. On the other hand, like most physicians, I was fearful of the transition to second-year resident—I would not only be making decisions on my own; I would also be responsible for guiding someone else's decision-making.

In addition to second year resident, the other overwhelming stages of medical training are the first year of fellowship and the first year as an attending physician. I didn't realize it then, though I know now, that every tough transition just requires mastery of new workflows and skillsets. Here are my strategies for surviving and thriving with each transition.

8.1.1 Second-Year Resident

Being a second-year resident worried me a lot. I would be the one nodding encouragingly as I reviewed the intern's work to ensure their evaluation and decision-making was accurate and complete. For the first time, there was no one to nod their head, pat my shoulder, and tell me that I did the right thing. While the attending physician would be there on morning rounds to ensure optimal patient care, it would be me, in the middle of the night, deciding if a patient was sick, or not sick, and guiding their diagnostic and treatment plan accordingly.

Of course, my confidence was sorely tested on my first call night as a second-year resident. I was the admitting resident at a small community hospital affiliated with the larger tertiary care center where I trained. A 90-year-old man came into the ED because he had tripped on his rug and fallen. He packed a little suitcase with toiletries and a change of clothes and presented to the hospital with a sore back. Given his age and laboratories consistent with dehydration, the intern and I admitted him to a non-telemetry unit and started intravenous fluids. I crawled into the bed in the call room after midnight, proud of myself. I had taught the intern clinical pearls about pneumonia and cholecystitis, not received any sidewise glances from seasoned nurses, and if all went well, I would have 4 h of sleep before morning rounds.

As it happened, I got 2 h of sleep. The code pager snapped me awake and as the on-call resident, it was my job to run the code. My intern was already at the bedside when I arrived, breathless, and the nurse was doing chest compressions. "What's the story?" I asked the intern, just as other residents had asked me when I was the scared-looking first-year resident. "We just admitted him!" she replied. It was the 90-year-old man who packed his suitcase after his mechanical fall, now with a PEA arrest.

After intubation and a few rounds of epinephrine and atropine, he had return of spontaneous circulation and was on his way to the ICU. Distraught, I asked the senior ICU resident what I missed; he just grunted, annoyed by the admission. I rotated back to the mothership a few days later and never found out what happened to the patient. Was it advanced heart block, VT, or a pulmonary embolism? A hemorrhagic stroke? Did I miss something? This case weighed on me and I found myself in the residency program director's office, talking it out. It was the embodiment of my worst fears, being the proximate cause of the patient's death. The worst part: I had no way of knowing if I was the cause.

My program director was incredible—a mentor for how to counsel trainees through tough cases. We reviewed the case together and it turned out the elderly gentleman had complete heart block, advanced conduction system disease, in the context of a restrictive cardiomyopathy (in retrospect, likely from cardiac amyloidosis). The best medical take-away: consider the patient's history and their clinical context when formulating a management plan: an elderly gentleman admitted after a fall deserves to be on telemetry monitoring even if he seems well enough to pack a suitcase before coming to the hospital and his only symptom is a sore back. The best mentoring take-away: lean on trusted physicians to talk through tough cases in a safe space.

I also feared being a second-year resident because I knew that it would be up to me to set the tone for the team. The medical students and interns would look to me for pearls of wisdom, humor, and morale-building. Could I be a charismatic and inspirational leader? Being captain of the high school math team probably didn't qualify as charismatic leadership experience. I doubted that I was up to the task, so I resorted to my usual practice: instead of worrying, I made a concrete action plan.

I envisioned rounding as a team leader, interjecting clinical pearls after every presentation. I resolved to prepare a pearl for every patient as I pre-rounded. That was a lofty goal, and sometimes I only offered a pearl on one or two patients on rounds: still, the act of preparation lessened my fear of being a leader.

8.1.2 First-Year Fellow

Being a first-year fellow and first-year attending are the two other scariest transitions. Being a first-year fellow is terrifying because residents and even attendings in other specialties ask you questions and think you know the answer (though for the most part, you don't know for sure—not yet). On one of my first weekend calls as a first-year cardiology fellow, a patient called because their peripherally-inserted central catheter had inadvertently pulled out about an inch. The patient had advanced heart failure and dobutamine was their lifeline. I spent a few minutes berating myself for my lack of experience before calling the attending physician on call. Of course, he knew what to do (send the patient to the emergency department for a chest x-ray to ensure appropriate positioning and re-dressing of the site, or new line placement if the positioning was not appropriate). It was stressful to be at the bottom of the learning curve again and not know the right answer. When this happens to you, don't waste time beating yourself up for not knowing what to do; make a plan to figure out what to do. Accept that you will need help: patience is one of the keys to experience.

8.1.3 Attending Physician

The uncertainty of being an attending physician follows these same themes, though the stakes are higher: now you are the one making the final call on life-and-death decisions. On the other hand, by the time you have become an attending physician, you have grown in maturity and experience. You have practiced making decisions with the safety net in place (why it's so important to be a Captain instead of a Waiter, as described later in this chapter.) You have established a group of trusted colleagues and mentors who can help you through the hard times. Equally as valuable, by the time you are an attending physician, you have collected countless medical students, interns, residents, and fellows under your wing. You are now a mentor yourself and you will learn from those you teach.

After years of training, it may be difficult to put your own experience into perspective. The first few coronary angiograms that I performed as an attending physician were nerve-wracking. Someone else was holding the needle, so while I had all the responsibility for the needle's trajectory, I had none of the authority. A hematoma over the femoral artery, dissection, pseudoaneurysm, or retroperitoneal bleed were all possible—and if they happened, it would be my responsibility to manage the complications and explain the ramifications to the patient and their family.

There are specific lessons to be quickly learned as a new attending physician guiding fellows in the cardiac catheterization laboratory. Adequately sedate the patient so that neither the few additional minutes the fellow requires to gain access nor the direction and commentary you provide to the fellow will alarm the patient. Pitch your tone as a calm, quiet, and matter-of-fact murmur for further reassurance. Offer precise and brief instruction on needle position. Gauge the fellow's skill by how well they follow instruction, how gently they probe with the needle, and how readily they cede access to the attending physician when they feel unsure.

As a brand-new attending, I dreaded having to take over when a fellow was unable to gain access. What if I were unable to gain access as well? In one of my first cases, the fellow struggled three times (my limit) and then handed the needle to me. Muscle memory, borne of the hundreds of cases I had performed myself as a fellow, took over and placement of the femoral arterial sheath was smooth and straightforward. I felt green and unsure, identifying with the fellow as I was only a few years ahead of her in training. However, I was no longer a green and unsure fellow. I should have realized that those years of training that separated us made all the difference. I had skills far exceeding hers, as I should, given my training. This was the turning point when I finally recognized that I had crossed a bridge from inexperience to experience.

I was still reeling from this revelation when my fellow and I started the next case. She had difficulty gaining access. I imagined what I would do differently if I were holding the needle. I directed her, calmly and precisely, to guide the needle laterally and deeper. I think I was more thrilled than she was when she successfully accessed the femoral artery. This mentorship showed me it was my time to lead. I did not need to be fearful because I was experienced.

As with most things in life, the anticipation of becoming a second-year resident, a first-year fellow, or an attending physician will be worse than reality. As a second-year resident, with a systematic approach and preparation, you can ensure that your intern leaves no stone unturned in the middle of the night. And as you grow more comfortable, you will find ways to insert teaching pearls into rounds and build morale (bringing brownies to rounds helps). As a fellow, you will have the safety net of an attending physician available to offer the right balance of autonomy and guidance as your experience grows. As an attending physician, you will have a coterie of trusted colleagues and mentors and keep them close, knowing where to turn for advice on clinical and professional quandaries.

I started out as a brand-new attending at an institution 3000 miles away from the institution where I was a fellow. While my new colleagues were very supportive, I had not yet established a network of local mentors, so I sent my clinical mentor from fellowship regular emails. I described interesting cases and asked his advice on challenging ones. Over the course of the first attending year, my emails went from weekly to monthly to every few months as I grew in experience and learned to trust and confide in my new colleagues.

At the completion of training, you will not undergo an instant transformation to seasoned physician. Though there will be flashes of insight, as when you successfully guide a fellow through vascular access, the feeling of experience will steal upon you slowly. As the years pass, you will reach out to some mentors more than others. The beauty of experience is that it continues to grow and there will always be someone who has more experience than you: someone you can learn from. No matter your career stage, you will always get by with a little help from your mentors.

In addition to the valuable sounding board of mentors, there are important strategies of teaching and learning to set you on your path of becoming an effective team leader.

8.2 Teaching

8.2.1 Streamline Rounds

Surgeons love to poke fun at internists for their interminable rounds, and with good reason. Rounds go on and on forever. The forever aspect of rounds is often spent on the data: the vital signs, physical examination, laboratory values, and imaging tests. A formal presentation may contain all these components. However, when a service is busy and the trainees are overwhelmed, shorter rounds will serve to optimize patient care and prioritize time for high-yield teaching.

How to streamline rounds? It starts with you, as the resident, fellow, or attending physician who will be running rounds, being prepared. Review all the objective data, from overnight orders to consultant notes to labs and imaging tests prior to rounds (see section on preparation in Chap. 7). If, as the team leader, you are aware of all the objective data, interns and medical students can skip the recitation of facts and proceed with a streamlined one-liner-and-straight-to-plan-by-system approach.

Some interns worry that important information will be missed. I reassure them that if a piece of objective data is important, it will be discussed in the assessment and plan, so reiteration just serves to maintain our reputation as ever-rounding internists.

Some interns worry that by speaking less, I will not be able to adequately evaluate their performance. I reassure them that shorter presentations that remain comprehensive and accurate are harder to master. Learning to speak less while saying more is a key skill for effective communication. When the intern concisely synthesizes the patient's presentation into a one-liner, the attending physician gains insight into their understanding and can critique and teach this important skill. The ability to identify and distill essential knowledge will serve trainees well throughout their career.

Besides teaching effective and efficient communication, streamlined rounds also provide trainees with enough time to get the real work done (entering orders, calling consultants). Most importantly, it will provide trainees with enough time to experience the joy of being a physician—they will have time to talk with their patients.

When an intern's presentation is going awry, should you interrupt them right away or wait until the end of their presentation to provide feedback? The answer depends on how far off course they have veered. Consider a patient admitted with decompensated heart failure. If the intern has made a critical error in the assessment, indicating that the patient is euvolemic warranting a transition to oral diuretic therapy when you know the patient is still volume-overloaded and requires intravenous diuresis, interrupt early. If the intern has the assessment right (volume overloaded) but the management wrong (furosemide 20 IV daily when you know the patient will only respond to a higher dose and frequency), wait until the end of the presentation to address the finer points of diuretic dose adjustments.

8.2.2 Encourage Debate

Physicians become great at reading patients' faces. You know just by a patient's still-ness, or eyelid twitch, or glance at the accompanying spouse, whether they agree or disagree with your plan. The same is true of trainees. Sometimes, trainees agree with your plan because they are convinced it is right. Other times, trainees go along with your plan just because you're the team leader. When faced with the latter situation, encourage debate.

A resident and I were caring for patient in cardiogenic shock. She was concerned that the patient was worsening and would soon require extracorporeal membrane oxygenation to maintain perfusion and preserve heart transplant candidacy. I explained why the patient's normal mentation, lack of tachycardia, and normal renal function indicated stability. I could tell she was uncomfortable, concerned that not urgently calling the cardiothoracic surgeon would result in the patient's demise.

I encouraged her to elaborate, and together we identified the source of our disagree-ment: she was concerned about the low thermodilution cardiac index despite esca-lating doses of inotropic support. We discussed the impact of severe tricuspid regur-gitation on the thermodilution cardiac index and the importance of incorporating multiple clinical parameters, including the Fick cardiac index and signs of perfu-sion, into the assessment of shock severity. I was grateful that she took an active role in the medical decision-making and had the courage to question mine. The ensuing discussion resulted in better understanding for her and better care for future patients.

Encouraging debate accomplishes many goals: (1) trainees learn that respectful disagreement is possible; (2) rounds become a safe space to learn without fear of being perceived as difficult or lacking aptitude; (3) trainees feel comfortable asking questions to deepen their understanding; and (4) team leaders confirm that their medical decision-making is appropriate, as the ability to explain a concept improves one's understanding of the concept. Respectful debate is a cornerstone of medical education.

When I sense a trainee doesn't agree with my plan, I'll say: "You seem uncon-vinced, so let's talk it out. Tell me what doesn't make sense so we can better under-stand the issue and provide the best care." What follows is a terrific discussion about the indications, risks, alternatives, and benefits of the chosen approach. Sometimes I convince the trainees and sometimes they convince me. Regardless, the patient receives optimal care, the trainees receive the best teaching, and the team leader has modeled respectful disagreement.

8.2.3 Create Captains-Claim the Role

I have observed that there are three kinds of trainees: the Toddler, the Waiter, and the Captain. The Toddler always wants their way and will not listen to reason when confronted with explanations of why their approach is incorrect. All inexperienced physicians have Toddler moments borne of fear. It is scary to admit that one does not, cannot, know everything about one's patients. As an intern, after reading about the differential diagnosis of hyponatremia, I was convinced that the syndrome of inappropriate antidiuretic hormone secretion from a brain tumor was the only correct diagnosis for my patient in heart failure with hyponatremia. Underlying my certainty was fear; I had to know everything or I wouldn't be able to save someone's life someday. As an attending physician, it's important to meet Toddlers with understanding, acknowledging the fear before you explain that their reasoning is wrong.

Waiters also fear not knowing everything, though their fear manifests as subservience rather than obstinance. At the start of a case in the cardiac catheterization laboratory, I asked the fellow, "What catheters should we use for this case?" The fellow replied, "Whatever catheters you want to use, Dr. Kittleson!" My response, to push him out of his Waiter comfort-zone: "What do YOU think we should use?" While his approach was polite and well-meaning, taking orders like a waiter is no way to learn. I wanted him to take charge and practice making decision.

Trainees may start out as Toddlers or Waiters and your goal as the team leader is to make them Captains. Your goal is to help them cross the bridge from inexperience to experience by replacing the fear with clear expectations and concrete action plans. With this system, all trainees can become Captains.

Captains help guide the ship. They present comprehensive assessments and plans, know the reason for every medication on the list, understand the trajectory of hospitalization, and can enumerate criteria for discharge. Every trainee can be a Captain if you provide expectations and offer a safe space to test out ideas. Providing expectations is key. Sometimes, the expectations may be explicit: "I expect you to not only provide me with a synthesis of the data, but your plan for the day."

Other times, the expectations may be implicit. A trainee might say, "The patient is volume overloaded. How much furosemide should we prescribe?" My response is always, "How much furosemide would YOU like to prescribe?" Do your best to not respond to basic management questions on rounds. Instead, ask the trainee to make a decision because future leaders need to practice decision-making. Indecision is dangerous. Patients may worry while doctors make a concrete action plan. Trainees learn to make a concrete action plan by practicing decision-making under the guidance of their attending physicians.

If the decision is wrong, it is the team leader's job to empower trainees to recover from errors in judgment and reassess the situation considering new information to achieve the right plan. For example, if the trainee responds to the question about diuretic dosing by recommending furosemide 20 mg IV daily and the day prior, the patient did not respond to this dose, point this out. Ask, "What were the I/Os on that dose yesterday? Are you satisfied with that diuresis? If not, what would be a better dose?" Guide the trainee to the right answer with a stepwise increase in relevant information. In the experienced physician's mind, the decision algorithm is straightforward and orderly; make it so for the trainee as well.

Sometimes, the erroneous decision is more deep-rooted and requires more than a quick readjustment in thinking. For example, for the trainee who thinks that a patient who is in heart failure is dry when the patient is actually wet, first recognize that assessment of volume status is challenging, even for experienced cardiologists. Next, discuss how you concluded that the patient was wet, not dry, and point out where the trainee strayed in their assessment. Third, ask the trainee if they are convinced and if not, discuss what further information may help better explain the issue. And finally, ask the trainee to revise their plan based on the new assessment. This method: (1) recognize the challenge, (2) walk through the thought process to identify the error, (3) ensure understanding, and (4) revise the thought process based on correct assumptions, allow trainees to feel comfortable making errors, readjusting their thinking, and making decisions.

8.2.4 Don't Micromanage

Medicine is an art, as well as a science. Sometimes a trainee will offer a plan that is not technically wrong though you just know, from your experience, that it is not the best one. Let's return to that patient in heart failure. The intern wants to prescribe furosemide 80 mg IV twice daily which is, ostensibly, a reasonable dose as the patient takes 40 mg twice daily at home. You have admitted this patient to the hospital before for decompensated heart failure and know that the patient will have a more robust response to a furosemide infusion of 20 mg/h. This knowledge is based on experience, not science, and there is no way the trainee could have intuited this.

One option is to change their plan. Another option is to tell them: "Your assessment and plan are sound. My experience from a prior hospitalization suggests a continuous infusion of furosemide would work better. Let's do this. Provide me with a contingency plan. If your approach does not yield X result in Y amount of time, you'll do Z." Then the trainee can think through the criteria for success as X, how long Y should be, and the alternative plan Z. They remain empowered to captain the ship and learn to pivot to contingencies when their plan proves ineffective or inferior.

8.2.5 Rejoice in Trainees' Successes

As the program director of the advanced heart failure and transplantation fellowship, I joke with my fellows that I am their program director for a year and their mom for life—except it's not really a joke. You spend so much time in the hospital that the staff is somewhere between a team and a family, complete with the requisite wise elders, eccentric aunts and uncles, and rebellious cousins. You care for each other as you together care for patients. I love receiving text messages with pictures of new houses and new babies. I love hearing about their honors and awards. Embrace the relationships you form with your trainees because their successes are your successes.

When your fellow performs a flawless endomyocardial biopsy on a heart transplant recipient, recognize that it was your mentorship that helped them to achieve this goal. The mentorship of medicine is an apprenticeship that traces back through generations of physicians. Your ability to mentor your fellows came from your mentors, and theirs from their mentors, and so on. Think about the countless physicians who molded you over the course of your training. As an experienced physician, you serve that role for every trainee you encounter. Little things can make a difference when you least expect it.

In *Cinema Paradiso*, projectionist and mentor Alfredo offers young Salvatore advice on pursuing his passion for filmmaking. Alfredo says, "Get out of here! Go back to Rome. You're young and the world is yours. I'm old. I don't want to hear you talk anymore. I want to hear others talking about you." That's the beauty of mentorship—expect your mentees to pay it forward instead of paying it back. Feedback may come years later or not at all; that does not minimize the importance of your role.

I have had trainees approach me years after graduation to thank me for mentorship. Sometimes it was the advocacy I provided to help them land their dream job. Other times, it is a small practice, like not trending the creatinine on rounds in a patient on dialysis. In ways large and small, you can make your trainees better physicians and there is nothing egotistical about rejoicing in your role.

Being a mentor means being part of a long thread of shared wisdom in medical education. Being a mentor also means a part of you remains a student. Always remember the importance of learning—you will take better care of your trainees and your patients if you do.

8.3 Learning

8.3.1 Look Things Up

You're never too important to look things up. No matter what stage you are in your career, you will have to look things up. Thank goodness for UpToDate, the physician's best friend. Active learning is better than passive learning, so if you find something you don't know, look it up right away. I treat patients with pericarditis, though not often, and therefore I can never remember the exact recommended dose/schedule of non-steroidal anti-inflammatory agents. I look it up every time and add the particulars to my note. Every time I look it up, the basic tenets are reinforced: NSAIDs are first-line, colchicine may be used if NSAIDs alone don't work, and steroids are associated with recurrent pericarditis. Placing new facts in context and reinforcing old ones is the best way to learn.

8.3.2 Know the Right Questions

As an inexperienced physician, I expended so much mental energy needlessly worrying about patients. When a patient was doing poorly, I worried that I was missing something. I worried that the patient would be doing better if a more experienced physician were caring for them. When a patient was doing well, I worried that they would worsen again and I would miss the signs. If I was caring for a patient—you name it, I worried about it. I spent as much energy worrying about what I didn't know as I did on caring for the patient.

I felt this way because I had not yet realized that no one, not even the most experienced physician, can know everything. I had not yet learned to replace worry with a plan. The key is not to know all the answers. The key is to know the right questions. If you ask the right questions, you can make a plan to find the answers.

When you're confused, figure out why. Are the patient's symptoms out of proportion to the benign results of the testing? I cared for a patient who presented with dyspnea on exertion. A stress test showed no ischemia and an echocardiogram showed normal left ventricular function, so I initially (mistakenly) assumed that his symptoms could not be cardiac in nature. I posited deconditioning and recommended a structured exercise program.

However, his symptoms progressed over the next few months and then I uncovered a physical exam finding that I had not observed at our initial encounter: an elevated jugular venous pressure. This sent me down the correct differential diagnosis of an infiltrative cardiomyopathy and the patient was ultimately diagnosed with AL amyloidosis and required heart transplantation.

In talking it over with a trusted colleague, I realized that I had not asked the right questions from the start. The patient's symptoms were out of proportion to the benign echocardiographic findings. Was it because the patient's symptoms were not cardiac in nature (as I had assumed) or because the echocardiogram was not adequate to assess for the source of his symptoms? In fact, the echocardiogram did show mildly increased left ventricular wall thickness which I had attributed to hypertension. If I had paid closer attention to the progressive nature of his symptoms and his jugular venous pressure, I might have paid closer attention to the increased left ventricular wall thickness and searched for an infiltrative cardiomyopathy sooner. When the patient's symptoms are at odds with objective findings, dig deeper. Review the differential diagnosis and the sources of false-negatives from the tests.

There are also instances when the objective findings are at odds with the patient's symptoms. In this case, the question is whether the diagnosis is correct. I cared for a patient with a longstanding nonischemic cardiomyopathy with progressive shortness of breath. When I met her, she was significantly hypoxic at rest requiring home oxygen and her chest x-ray showed bilateral diffuse fluffy infiltrates, which didn't match her physical examination which was consistent with euvolemia. Her presentation felt more pulmonary than cardiac and it turns out that she had interstitial lung disease in addition to a nonischemic cardiomyopathy as the cause of her decompensation.

Finally, there are situations where a given course of treatment is not having the desired effect, which then leads to a questioning of the diagnosis. For a patient with decompensated heart failure, this can be when diuresis to treat volume overload results in progressive renal dysfunction or hypotension. This is either happening because the patient remains volume overloaded with cardiogenic shock or because the patient is not wet in the first place. The key in this situation is knowing how to obtain the right answer: get more information from a pulmonary artery catheter.

So, when it comes to asking the right question, think to yourself: (1) is the patient sicker than the test results; (2) are the tests more abnormal than the patient; (3) are the treatments not having the desired effect? Then, delve deeper into your differential diagnosis to determine the pitfalls of the diagnostic testing and involve the appropriate consultants if you cannot answer the questions on your own (more on interpretation of test results in Chap. 5).

8.3.3 Experience Trumps Education

Your mentors don't have to be physicians and they don't have to be older than you. It was a fellow who was my mentor when he first introduced me to Twitter. I had more experience in medicine and he had more experience in social media.

I am so grateful for experienced technologists in the cardiac catheterization laboratory. When I was a fledgling attending physician having difficulty engaging an aberrant coronary artery, an experienced technologist would often stand beside me, ready with a wet gauze or flush, and whisper, "Maybe you should try this catheter?" Thank goodness for the gracious and generous assistance of the unsung heroes of the medical profession: the experienced intensive care unit nurses, respiratory therapists, pharmacists, cardiac catheterization laboratory technologists, and so many others who have seen it all. These experienced members of the medical team were honing their craft while you were studying for the medical school entrance exams; listen, learn, and use their experience to provide optimal patient care.

8.4 Feedback

As a fellow, we received anonymous written feedback from the attending physicians at the end of every rotation. I could intuit based on the timing of the written review and my rotation schedule which attending physician had written it. Most of mine was complimentary though there was one attending physician in the CCU who wrote, "Michelle is overly controlling and prescriptive of the housestaff." It's amazing that over two decades later, I can recite this negative comment verbatim and remember who gave it to me. There is no role for unkindness in medicine. Unkindness increases fear and keeps trainees locked in inexperience.

While his feedback might have been true (I had not yet mastered the art of not micromanaging the trainees under my care), it was unhelpful in so many ways. First, it was not timely, having occurred weeks after my Napoleonic behavior had occurred. Second, it was not specific. Was it okay when I interrupted the intern who was planning to start heparin with a bolus in a patient with a recent intracranial bleed without first consulting neurology? Or was it wrong when I haggled with the resident regarding the duration of antibiotics for a ventilator-associated pneumonia? Third, it did not provide context: to make the comment less hurtful and more useful, it would have been helpful to know how changing my behavior would impact patient care. Was I so unpleasant to work with that trainees felt they did not have a safe space to test their nascent medical knowledge? Fourth, there were no strategies for improvement: should I have waited until the end of rounds to provide guidance rather than interrupting throughout? Finally, the attending physician did not circle back to assess my progress, as by the time I received the feedback, the rotation had ended.

Perhaps because the negative feedback was provided without context, I thought of it often; the impact of negative comments lingers longer than that of the positive ones. Ironically, the attending physician who made this comment was one of the most controlling and prescriptive attendings around. His rounds were not a safe space encouraging discussion; fellows barely said a word on rounds. Considering the source, I still wonder what I did to deserve this negative evaluation and what I could have done better. Having felt the sting of this feedback, I try to be better.

The moral of the story is not to avoid negative feedback. The moral is to make this feedback constructive instead of destructive. Inexperienced physicians often confess to me that offering feedback can be nerve-wracking because they do not want to be perceived as "mean." Take personal feelings out of this professional interaction. Have high standards because lives are at stake. Don't be unkind, or rude, or thoughtless. Consider this stepwise process below to offer concrete, objective, and actionable feedback. Sometimes it's hard to know exactly what to say, and thus I offer concrete examples based on specific effective feedback that I've given or received.

8.4.1   Be Timely

Feedback should be given as soon as possible. Imagine a trainee admits an immuno-suppressed patient with urosepsis and the patient has a history of recurrent urinary tract infections with antibiotic-resistant organisms. The trainee starts an antibiotic and calls the infectious disease consultant who has cared for the patient on prior admissions. Though the consultant leaves a note late that night recommending a change in antibiotics, no one on the team reviews the note until the next morning and the antibiotic order is delayed by 12 h. Who is at fault? The consultant could have communicated the recommendations directly to the primary team. That does not release the resident from their responsibility. The resident should have checked the chart and followed up on consultant's recommendations.

The feedback should occur on morning rounds, not 2 weeks later at the end of the rotation. It does not need to be long or drawn-out. It can be simply, "It's essential to review the chart before you leave for the day and sign out any outstanding issues, including consultant recommendations. If you do this, the patient will not have a potentially significant delay in administration of appropriate antibiotics."

8.4.2 Be Specific

Describe specific instances when care could have been improved. One of my litmus tests is to ask a trainee the indication of a medication on a patient's list (see Art of the Oral Presentation in Chap. 2). This isn't just an exercise in identifying Captains; it illustrates an important tenet of optimal patient care. If a trainee cannot explain the reason for a medication, I will explain exactly why it is so important: "If the patient is on ferrous sulfate and you do not know when it was prescribed or when iron studies were last checked, then you may be continuing a potentially unnecessary medication."

8.4.3 Provide Context

Of course, it should be obvious that the only reason you, as the attending physician, are taking the time and trouble to provide feedback is because you want to make your trainees better physicians. Trainees may not realize that it requires less time, effort, and energy to tell them they are doing a great job than to critically dissect their performance. Emphasize: "You are going to be a good physician who cares about your patients no matter what. Feedback is part of becoming a great physician. When you tell me that the patient has a history of PTLD, know what that acronym stands for. Build your knowledge in context."

8.4.4 Offer Strategies to Improve

There are actionable and concrete habits a trainee can adopt to become more thorough and detail-oriented. Willpower, ego, and aptitude will only take a trainee so far—it is up to you, as the experienced physician, to provide your trainees with a system. Share specific strategies: "You forgot to check the patient's urine output before you left for the day, and this was not signed out to the overnight resident. If you had a system of checkboxes for your to-do list, whether on a piece of paper or your phone, this would not have fallen through the cracks. Let's go over your to-do list at the end of rounds to ensure the small but important details are not forgotten."

8.4.5 Check in to Assess Progress

There is nothing more satisfying that seeing a trainee improve as the rotation progresses, starting out with wandering presentations full of extraneous information presented in a disorganized manner that transform into clean, concise, and comprehensive outlines of the patient's current state and trajectory. When a trainee begins the rotation with plans that consist of a recitation of data and ends the rotation with plans that include action items and contingencies, you have succeeded. You, as the attending physician, will have provided key habits and a system that will serve them well for a lifetime in medicine.

8.4.6 Positive Feedback is Important Too

Just because it's feedback doesn't mean it has to be critical. I was asked by the hospital's peer review committee to review the records of a pregnant patient who had passed away shortly after delivery from a polymorphic VT arrest to determine if there had been deficiencies in her care. In reviewing the chart, I could not grasp the timeline because everyone had copied forward the initial note which offered little detail. Did she had a peripartum cardiomyopathy or a reduced ejection fraction from myocardial stunning post resuscitation? Did she have a prolonged QT interval on ECG prior to administration of QT-prolonging medication? I was ready to give up when I encountered a beautifully organized note that outlined the patient's course perfectly. Finally, thanks to this note, I could accurately evaluate the patient's quality of care.

When I reached the end of this note, I discovered that it had been authored by a former fellow. I was so proud. I emailed him to let him know that his note had been spectacular and helped me to provide optimal patient care. He responded right away, with thanks, and to let me know that my email was well-timed: it had been a hard week as a new attending physician and my email had lifted his spirits.

One lesson here is to write clear notes (explained in The Art of the Note in Chap. 2). The other lesson is that positive feedback is essential. There is a right time to deliver negative feedback; there is never a wrong time to dole out the positive kind.

Provide positive feedback to the trainees in front of the patients. For example, if the fellow does a phenomenal job outlining the case of a complicated patient to the Heart Transplant Selection Committee, I will tell the patient, on rounds with the fellow, that it was the fellow's hard work that contributed to his acceptance on the heart transplant waiting list.

Provide positive feedback to patients about referring physicians. As a heart failure and transplant cardiologist, I see many patients with cardiac amyloidosis. This is an important diagnosis to make as there are specific disease-directed therapies to help people feel better and live longer. However, the diagnosis cannot be made with routine testing; you must order specific tests with the diagnosis in mind. When a patient presents to me for management after the diagnosis has been made by the general cardiologist, I make sure to give the referring cardiologist credit. It gives the patient the appropriate faith in their primary cardiologist and gives the primary cardiologist well-deserved recognition for their diagnostic acumen and clinical judgment.

The key attributes of an experienced physician are honesty and humility: you can exhibit both as you provide positive feedback about your trainees and colleagues to patients. Always provide credit where credit is due. Medicine is a team sport; stay humble and support your team.

8.5 Lead with Kindness

8.5.1 Protect Your Team

There are many fine things about being an attending physician. At the top of the list is the fact that people will act respectfully just because you are the attending physician. This became very clear to me during my training. As a fellow, I had to round on a patient who only wanted to see a particular attending physician. When I entered her room, she would greet me with, "So, you're Dr. X's flunkie today?" I never protested, though the moniker rankled. One day, I was rounding with her favorite attending physician when she turned to him and said, "So, when do you change flunkies?".

He was renowned for his calm and kind bedside manner, and remained calm and kind. He told her that while she was sick and tired of being in the hospital, there was never an excuse to be rude. He explained that I was assisting him in her care because I was qualified and because he trusted me. He concluded by telling her that to call someone who had spent 4 years in college, 4 years in medical school, 3 years in internal medicine residency training, 3 years in general cardiology training, and was now in advanced training a "flunkie" was mean and counterproductive. She shrugged, changed the subject, and never called me a flunkie again. This interaction occurred in the days before patient reviews. Given the chance, would she have vented her frustration in an anonymous telephone survey? (Not that I would have read it; more on that in Chap. 13).

As a trainee, you receive so many slights, large and small. These slights build up to the point that you begin to accept and ignore them. When a mentor takes the time to defend you, you realize that you have not ignored the slights after all. Rather, you have buried the hurt. As he politely explained to her why her words were hurtful and unacceptable, I felt the warm glow of someone standing up for me. His actions were also a revelation. First, you can have a conflict with a patient, and do so respectfully so that the patient-physician bond is preserved. Second, you never forget how awful it is to feel slighted and how wonderful it feels to be validated and defended. And finally, when you defend your team members, you inspire them to return the favor when they are in a position of power.

When you witness a trainee being disrespected, say something. Sometimes they're disrespected by patients and other times by staff or other physicians. Handle these situations differently. Patients may be in pain, scared, anxious, confused, and stressed out, so approach the situation with that understanding in mind. Be a calm and kind role model. Start by expressing how hard it is to have multiple team members with different messages. Promise to do your best to streamline communication and go through what behavior is acceptable (fear and sorrow) and what is not (anger and rudeness)—more on this in Chap. 9.

When it is a staff member who is rude, approach their supervisor or manager first for advice on how to handle the situation. Counsel the trainee if their behavior was inappropriate (taking too long to answer a call or responding in a snarky fashion) and ask the supervisor if they will address the situation with their staff member. It is a tricky thing to reprimand someone who works in a parallel management structure. In my experience, approaching the staff member's supervisor for direction is the most effective strategy.

If it is another physician, use a similar tactic. If it is a trainee in another program, discuss the situation with their program director. If the rudeness stems from a fellow attending physician, their seniority relative to your own will dictate the approach. When I was a junior attending physician, I would often seek out the counsel of a senior mentor. When I would email a clear description of the issue and problem, I would copy my senior colleague, already apprised of the situation, on the email. By doing so, I had a senior colleague to support me as I strove to provide optimal patient care.

I find an email like this works best: "When you rounded on Mr. X yesterday, you told the resident that his plan was rubbish and he needed to read more before asking you for advice. While I agree that the resident should read up on the topic, it would be best to avoid insulting them as you offer advice. Let me know if you would like to chat directly." Whether the rudeness stems from a patient, staff member, or physician, the approach is the same: use understanding, give a little, ask a little.

Rudeness is a sign of inexperience, regardless of how long you have been practicing medicine. You may command fear—though never respect –with rudeness. The experienced physician will be calm and assertive, never rude, even when delivering critical feedback—even to patients.

8.5.2   Don't Just Make the Offer, Make a Plan

When I was a junior attending physician, weekend calls were brutal, with one attending physician on call from Friday night at 5 PM to Monday morning at 8 AM. I would divide the call mentally into 5 12-h shifts (though it was a bit longer, I know) and focus on surviving each block. There would be at least 30 patients to round on in the hospital and calls from patients, nurses, and physicians at all hours of the day and night. There were trips back to the hospital in the middle of the night to see consults. In short, it was exhausting both physically and mentally, and early in my career, the mental stress was the worst. I was always anticipating a call that I would not know how to handle. The Monday morning after a call weekend was often my happiest time. Even as I dragged myself through that post-call week, heavy with the accumulated exhaustion of that call weekend, I always felt the relief of knowing it was the longest stretch until I was on weekend call again.

Imagine my chagrin when I discovered, due to changes in coverage, I had to be on call two weekends in a row. I did not complain about it, though I experienced a significant amount of anticipatory dread as the first call weekend approached. One of my senior colleagues noticed that I was scheduled to be on call two weekends in a row and offered to take the Sunday afternoon/night of my first call weekend. Of course, I said no: I was proud and wanted to show him that I was a hard worker and team player. When I said no, he just smiled and said, "Too bad, because I already told the answering service to route all calls to me starting at 4 PM Sunday through Monday morning. Have a glass of wine and relax." And so I did—two glasses, actually. He taught me that if you really want to help someone, you don't just offer to help, you make a plan they cannot refuse.

Because of this kindness shown to me, I try to do that for others. Sometimes, when the team is swamped, I will not just offer to write some notes, I'll let them know which patients I've assigned myself. Specific plans are hard to refuse and making plans takes the burden off the person who needs the help.

8.6 Final Thoughts

Being a leader does not come naturally to most people, and that's okay. The secret to great leadership is establishing the importance of a shared mission and the mission in medicine is optimal patient care. If you are motivated by a desire to provide optimal patient care, you will create a safe space of respect and kindness where others can do so. Becoming a leader takes time and experience—but all the experience does not have to be your own. You will observe leaders who are skillful and others who are not. With the help of these role models and mentors, you will fashion your leadership style. You will establish systems of teaching, learning, and feedback that will benefit you, your trainees, and your patients throughout your career.

Chapter 9
The Tough Conversations

Great science doesn't save lives. The correct equation is: great science plus effective implementation equals lives saved. Effective implementation requires clear communication and trust. As a trainee, I honed my style of communication by observing my residents, fellows, and attending physicians, both those who communicated well and those who communicated poorly. I also learned by observing the impact of my words on my patients. My children helped too. Toddlers will challenge your patience. They teach you when to stand your ground and when to concede and how to communicate with someone in the midst of an emotional maelstrom. Managing emotions, whether those of your loved ones or your patients, is an art.

The first and most obvious rule of communication is to avoid medical jargon. After spending what seems like forever mastering medical terminology, trainees often have difficulty leaving this terminology behind when talking with patients. Most patients have no idea what "renal failure" or "febrile" means. When you speak with a patient, pretend that you are speaking with a non-medical parent or friend. You would find ways to explain their medical condition without resorting to complex terminology; do the same for your patients. As an attending physician, when you observe trainees communicating with patients, point out (afterwards, not in front of the patient), when they used medical terminology that the patient probably did not understand.

I worked with a wonderful trainee who told the patient that her laboratories showed "stage 4 CKD from hypertension." When he used this phrase on rounds, I was proud of him because he had accurately defined and stratified her medical condition and identified the underlying contributing diagnosis. When he used this phrase at the patient bedside, the patient's eyes grew wide with fear (stage 4 sounds bad!) and confusion (CKD? Hypertension?). I felt badly for the patient. I felt worse when she asked, "Do I have cancer? Stage 4?" It took some extra time to explain the classification scheme of chronic kidney disease and address her greatest fears: there was no cancer, her kidneys were not in imminent danger of failing, she was not going to need dialysis anytime soon, and there were strategies to preserve and maintain her kidney function.

When we debriefed after rounds, I asked how he would explain this patient to a nonmedical friend. I could see the lightbulb go off in his head. The next day, he explained diverticulitis clearly and simply to another patient, offering relevant medical facts and a concrete action plan. When we left the room, the patient was grateful and reassured. This intern had taken another step across the bridge from inexperience to experience, improving his communication skills by avoiding jargon, a technique that would benefit his future patients.

9.1   The Emotion Behind the Question

There is often an emotion behind the question, and it's important to address both the question and the emotion behind it. First you must listen to the patient—and I mean really listen. I care for many patients with heart failure who are stable with minimal symptoms for years. Some reach a tipping point when their symptoms progress and they require additional testing and adjustment in medications. When I recommend a new medication, there will often be a flurry of questions: what are the side effects, is it safe with all my other medications, will I have to take this medication for the rest of my life? As a physician, you must address these questions and you must also address the emotions behind them: Can I trust you? Am I going to be okay?

9.1.1   Can I Trust You?

How do you let a patient know that they can trust you? Sometimes, I explain this explicitly: "My only agenda is to help you feel better and live longer." Other times, you show patients that they can trust you through the effort you have devoted to advanced preparation. Demonstrate, through the time and trouble you've taken to sort out the details of their complex medical history, that you will provide optimal care.

You may also show patients that they can trust you by the non-medical questions you ask, focusing on their childhood, family, and work because you care about them as more than a collection of diagnoses. The effort you expend on advanced preparation and on learning the non-medical details is never wasted. The former is essential and the latter especially will bring you joy, strengthen your bond, and provide the trust essential for optimal patient care.

Francis Peabody said, "... the reward is to be found in that personal bond which forms the greatest satisfaction of the practice of medicine. One of the essential qualities of the clinician is interest in humanity, for the secret of the care of the patient is in caring for the patient." Show interest in your patient's humanity and they will know that you care about them.

9.1.2 Am I Going to Be Okay?

When a heart failure patient requires medication adjustments due to worsening symptoms, they may ask about side effects and drug interactions. What they really want to know is if they are going to be okay. How do you let patients know that they're going to be okay? You can ask patients what their greatest fear is and other times, from experience, you may intuit it. Either way, the next step is to address the greatest fear by (1) empowering patients to control what they can and (2) helping them accept what they can't. Put a voice to their fears, offer tempered optimism, and manage expectations.

For the patient with worsening heart failure, I discuss the greatest fear of needing a heart transplant. I empower them to control what they can: being on the optimal medications to preserve heart function, quality of life and survival, and avoiding behaviors that compromise heart function like use of alcohol or illicit substances. Then, I explain that whether they will someday need a heart transplant is impossible to predict and out of their control. I encourage them to focus on what they can control (optimal medications and lifestyle) and to accept what they can't (the possibility of a heart transplant 10 years hence).

Help the patient to focus on what they can control and accept what they cannot. This strategy will allow you to address the emotion behind the question and successfully navigate tough conversations with patients. Here are my strategies for specific tough scenarios you may encounter—strategies that will help you confront the strong emotions and focus your efforts on providing the best care.

9.2 The Patient Who is Angry and Frustrated

When I was a third-year medical student, a patient reduced me to tears. She was an elderly woman with cancer who had undergone extensive surgery including removal of tissue from her leg for grafting to her face and neck. The senior resident asked me to remove the leg sutures during rounds. My resident demonstrated the first few and then left me to finish the rest. As I gingerly snipped each suture, the patient screamed insults: I was incompetent, the nurses were rude, the hospital food was making her sick. I soldiered on, carefully removing the seemingly hundreds of sutures running up her leg, because my resident told me to. By the time I rejoined the team to finish rounds, I was in tears.

This encounter still bothers me, and not just because I embarrassed myself by crying on surgical rounds. Rather, I'm still bothered because I never figured out what the patient was really angry about. Was it pain from the suture removal? Was it worry about her prognosis? Was it because her family rarely visited?

I tried to hold back my tears and the surgical residents regarded me as they would a tumor that starts spurting blood as it's excised: fear mixed with horror. The senior resident told me not unkindly that I had to "get it together." She explained that there would be many more angry and frustrated patients in my future and that their emotions weren't personal. She was right, of course. I was not the source of the patient's anger and frustration, simply an available target. While it's true that I needed to "get it together," there are more specific strategies that may be helpful for working with a patient who is angry.

Through the lens of experience, I know not to take any powerful emotion personally (and that applies to praise as much as anger). Here are my strategies for dealing with a patient who is angry and frustrated.

9.2.1   Protect Yourself

While the patient is your top priority, it is important to protect yourself. I was in no physical danger from this weak, elderly, hospitalized woman, though her stream of invective was hurtful and distracting. If this happened now, I would explain that her abuse was not acceptable, ask if she wanted to talk about why she was angry and frustrated, and if she continued to spout insults and slurs, leave the room. I would return later when she was hopefully calmer to complete the suture removal. The first rule of an angry and frustrated patient: there is reasonable anger and there is unreasonable anger. When faced with unreasonable anger: threats of violence, abusive language, or fear for your safety, separate yourself from the situation immediately. Whether you return on your own, or with staff including security, depends on the situation. First and foremost, however, protect yourself when you feel threatened.

Unreasonable anger happens all too often, as we know from reading terrible stories in the press. In the day-to-day life of a physician, reasonable anger is more common. The senior surgical resident was right: though it's rarely ever about you, it's still your responsibility to absorb, direct, and defuse.

We have all succumbed to the emotional overload of reasonable anger and frustration. When we are overwhelmed by fear, we can all blow our top, and the life-and-death stakes of the hospital heighten every emotion. Be empathetic when strong emotion short-circuits reason and judgment. There is no use meeting anger and frustration with reason and logic. As anyone in a close relationship knows, when faced with strong emotion, you must understand the issue before you attempt to fix it.

Nothing inflames an already agitated loved one more than, "You need to calm down." Why? Because attempting to make the problem go away without first trying to understand it tells the other person that either you don't care or you can't be bothered. Your intentions are good. Make sure your actions are as well. And the start of good actions is listening.

9.2.2   Step 1: Listen

When dealing with an angry and frustrated patient, one who is emotional without raising their voice, hurling abuse, or threatening physical violence, just listen. And when I say listen, I mean... listen. What are they angry and frustrated about? Because I deal with many patients in stressful life-and-death situations, I can often anticipate the source of their anger and frustration: they can't have breakfast, their breakfast is late, they need to go to an inpatient rehabilitation facility, or they cannot go home until tomorrow. These are not minor issues for patients who are sick, scared, anxious, stressed out, and/or in pain—they may be the proverbial straw that broke the camel's back. At times, I rush the listening process because I have heard them before.

I may cut into step 2 (reflect the emotions to show understanding) before a patient is done telling me why they are angry and frustrated. This is not a good idea. Interjecting is rude and (as I have learned through experience) results in more anger and frustration. You cannot go through the motions. You must listen to the patient and let them have their say. Listening might feel like it takes forever; it doesn't. Give the patient a few minutes of your time to show them you respect their feelings.

9.2.3   Step 2: Reflect

At some point, the patient will have said what they needed to say, felt that you have heard them, and then they will stop. Now, it's your turn. Reflect on the source of the anger and frustration. Even when out of proportion—patient threatening to leave the hospital against medical advice because breakfast was late—there is always a kernel of truth. Identify—and empathize with—the kernel of truth.

For a hospitalized patient, everything is out of their control. That feels scary, and patients have the right to be upset. Facing and accepting this unavoidable loss of control is important. Be honest with an angry and frustrated patient. Put yourself in their shoes: "I cannot imagine how stressful it is to be stuck in the hospital, being whisked away for procedures with little notice, not knowing when you can leave the hospital, not knowing where you are going to go when you leave. It feels like there is so little that you can rely on or look forward to in the hospital, and I can see why not getting your breakfast on time is the last straw." Put yourself in the patient's position and imagine what it feels to lose control of everything, from your health to your future to what and when you can eat. If you see the situation from your patient's perspective, you will not be shocked or surprised by their strong emotions—and your understanding is an essential component of optimal patient care.

When you get it right, when you have understood the situation and shown the patient that you understand, the look of relief on the patient's face is extraordinary. Most people do not want to be angry or unreasonable. However, when stressed, hurt, and frustrated, it may seem like there is no other way to be heard. Meet anger and frustration with empathy instead of judgment. When you identify with patients instead of chastising patients, you will feel their relief and you will make a connection. They will know they made the right decision to trust you with their feelings and they will be open to your strategies to fix the problem.

9.2.4   Step 3: Make a Concrete Action Plan

Once the strong emotion has been vented, processed, and understood, the next step is to figure out what can be done differently. There are some issues that you cannot control: procedures will happen at all hours of the day and night in the hospital without warning, patients will be too weak to go straight home and will require a stay at inpatient rehabilitation, and breakfast will be late. Perhaps the nurse and the radiology department can coordinate timing of tests and prepare the patient. Maybe the patient can have a supply of snacks available in their room when breakfast is late. Sometimes, nothing can be fixed. In my experience, just showing that you care and understand and are trying to help makes all the difference in the world.

9.2.5   Step 4: Circle Back

When strong emotions have been vented, the patient may feel embarrassed or ashamed, even though they shouldn't. Circle back later to check in and to thank them for sharing their concerns with you. Hospitalization creates an awful power differential: lying down versus standing, hospital gown+underwear versus clothes + shoes, no shower in days vs washed hair and fresh make-up. As best you can, minimize the power differential. There are small ways to minimize it, like by sitting at the bedside instead of standing. There are big ways too, like by thanking the patient for being honest with you when they are upset. Make sure patients understand that while you cannot make everything perfect, you will do your best to make things better.

9.3   Leaving Against Medical Advice

Angry and frustrated patients may leave against medical advice (AMA) or threaten to. Do your best to avoid discharging patients AMA because the label will follow the patient forever. If you can, protect them from suffering the consequences of emotional decision-making. Future chart readers will peg the patient an uncooperative and antagonistic. Before resorting to this harmful characterization, strive to understand their situation.

I cared for a patient admitted with progressively worsening heart failure. The plan was diuresis and an inpatient transplant evaluation. His outpatient cardiologist explained that he would probably be in the hospital for at least week for the evaluation, or longer if he was deemed unstable enough to wait in the hospital until transplantation.

I met him for the first time as weekend coverage on a Saturday morning, two days into his admission. He was responding well to a continuous infusion of furosemide along with dopamine to augment diuresis. I expected to have a brief check-in where I reiterated the plan and he nodded politely, already familiar with said plan.

I was shocked when he told me that he was leaving the hospital that afternoon. His childcare plans had fallen through, and he needed to be home. My heart broke when he explained the details: he was a widower with a teenage son. His wife had passed away unexpectedly a few years prior. The boy, now in high school, was still grappling with his mother's death as he faced his father's illness. While his father needed a heart transplant evaluation, his son needed him more.

While ostensibly he was leaving against my medical advice, I understood his predicament. I fashioned an outpatient oral diuretic regimen, though I feared he would soon be back in the hospital. I explained that a delay of a few weeks in listing him was reasonable, so that he could better plan for a longer hospital stay. I warned that a longer delay could jeopardize his transplant candidacy as he would risk of progressive deterioration and damage to his other organs. We compromised on discharge home with outpatient follow-up in a few days and a plan for readmission in a few weeks.

I purposely did not document that he left the hospital against medical advice because when those words appear in the chart, the "noncompliant" chart rumor follows patients forevermore. I knew, from prior experience, that when a label of "noncompliant" appears in a patient's chart, there could be significant implications for their future heart transplant candidacy. I did not want this patient, with his reasonable predicament, to have any potential barriers obstructing his road to life-saving therapies. I chose consensus over contention because I understood his plight. Make a partnership, not an adversarial relationship, your goal. Consider the impetus for a patient's behavior, not just the outcome.

I am relieved that we achieved consensus. I maintained his trust, and he returned to the hospital a few weeks later, prepared for a long stay. Just because you're right medically doesn't mean your plan is best for the patient. Meet desperation with patience and compassion. Think long and hard before you blame a patient and discharge them against medical advice.

9.4 The Patient Who Takes Too Long

Sometimes patients get lost telling their story. They become mired in minutiae to avoid painful facts, or they get mired in emotions and lose the thread of the story. They may be worried, flustered, or unsure of which details are important. A question about how long they have had chest pain may start with a story of their birth: they were told they had a heart murmur though you know, after review of their records, they have no congenital heart condition.

The first question to ask yourself is: are they really taking too long? Physicians give patients 11 s on average to explain the reasons for their visit before interrupting (Singh et al 2019). Are you guilty of this? Sometimes that's okay; guidance can help. Other times, it's important to allow the patient to get the story out in their own way so they can share what's important to them.

There are strategies you can use to guide the discussion and help the patient reach the heart of the matter (no pun intended). First, preparation is key because if you have reviewed relevant history in advance, you can skip descriptions of past medical history and focus only on current symptoms. I will say, "I have had a chance to review your chart and am familiar with your prior history [*insert summary here*]. Let's start with how you're feeling right now." Patients appreciate your preparation and understand where to start the story.

Other times, despite guidance, patients still have difficulty collecting their thoughts. In this situation, I find the phrases, "We don't have a lot of time and I want to use it as efficiently as possible" or "If I may interject" are helpful to gently guide the conversation to the high-yield and relevant information. Sir William Osler said, "Listen to the patient, he will tell you the diagnosis." He was right—to a point. Know when it is acceptable, even preferable, to guide the patient and how to do it kindly and respectfully.

9.5 The Patient Who Disagrees with You

My tenth-grade French teacher would put the class through an exercise he called "*Me convaincre*" [*Convince me*]. He started with a basic premise like "I don't believe the sky is blue" and then the student had to convince him (in French) that the sky was in fact blue. The purpose of this routine was to teach us to think in a foreign language (much as medical school teaches us to think in the language of medicine).

We would practice a wide range of French grammar and vocabulary and it would always end with an exasperated student because our otherwise flexible and easygoing teacher would hold mulish sway to his obviously wrong stance. When the student would finally give up ("*J'abadonne!*"), the teacher would laugh and offer a piece of advice that, unlike most of my French grammar, I never forgot: There are some people you will never convince, and the trick is knowing when to cut your losses.

This is often true in medicine, and medical decision-making is rarely as clear-cut as the color of the sky. Patients will disagree with your management plans, and the key in any disagreement is to (1) figure out the source of the difference of opinion; (2) offer your perspective; and (3) in possession of all the medical facts, allow the patient to make their decision. (This method is especially useful in the medically and emotionally fraught decision-making surrounding Covid 19—more on this in Chap. 13).

9.5.1 Step 1: Identify the Problem

Sometimes the disagreement is over something minor. The patient has an elevated blood pressure for the second time in a few months. You recommend blood pressure medications. The patient responds, "No, I don't want to take them. Why do I even need them?" The next step, of course, is to figure out why they don't want to take blood pressure medications. Sometimes it's an aversion to pills, the experience of a friend or neighbor with a reaction to a medication, not believing that hypertension is a problem in the first place, or meeting fear of having a medical diagnosis with denial.

Other times, the disagreement is over something major. The patient has advanced heart failure, you recommend a heart transplant evaluation, and the patient declines. Sometimes their disagreement stems from fear and denial, disbelief that their heart is weak enough to warrant transplant consideration, or a friend's bad experience with heart surgery.

While stakes may be vastly different, in both cases you need to uncover the source of the disagreement so you can best address it with the relevant medical facts—in other words, figure out the emotion behind the action.

9.5.2 Step 2: Emphasize the Shared Mission and Medical Facts

Never turn a disagreement with a patient into a win-lose situation because it isn't. If you convince the patient to agree with you, it's not that you have won and they have lost. If the patient does not come around, it's not that you have lost and they have won. Rather, the conversation is an attempt to find consensus towards a shared goal.

If a patient disagrees with my assessment on the need for blood pressure medication, I start by emphasizing that we both want the same thing for the patient: a long and happy life. I explain that untreated high blood pressure increases the risk of heart failure, kidney failure, and stroke. I remind the patient that my goal is to prevent the patient from ever experiencing one of these problems, and the best way to do so is to control blood pressure through healthy diet, exercise, and medications.

Depending on the specific source of disagreement, I may explain that hypertension often doesn't have symptoms and that the lack of symptoms doesn't make it any less serious. I explain that it may take a few months to find the right combination of medications that controls blood pressure with minimum side effects. I contrast the inconvenience of taking a daily pill to the devastation of a stroke. I explain that while it's natural to not want to get older and have high blood pressure, it's best to treat a problem rather than ignore it and pretend it will go away.

Heart transplantation is a more serious intervention, though the process is the same: emphasize the shared goal, medical facts, and consequences of their decision. Then, offer more detailed medical information targeted to the patient's specific fears and concerns.

9.5.3   Step 3: Allow the Patient to Make Their Own Decision

I usually end the discussion with: "You're the boss of your body, and I'm your medical consultant. I need to make sure that I've given you all the facts, and then you can make the decision that's right for you. Tell me how I can help you make your decision." At this point, some patients thank me for the careful explanation, and we decide on a treatment plan. Other patients remain unwavering in their opinion that high blood pressure is not a problem or heart transplantation is not indicated. At that point, I remember the words of my tenth-grade French teacher and agree to disagree. When the stakes are really high, though, I won't stop there: I'll offer a second opinion.

While a conversation about elevated blood pressure and the need for medications can occur again over the ensuing few months without significant harm, other issues like advanced heart failure are time sensitive. I evaluated a patient with hypertrophic cardiomyopathy, referred by his primary cardiologist due to worsening shortness of breath. There were many red flags that heralded poor prognosis for him: progressive symptoms, falling ejection fraction, worsening renal function, rising diuretic requirement, and reduced maximal consumption on cardiopulmonary exercise stress testing. When I explained all of this, he remained hesitant. I knew that he did not have months to years to ponder the decision; a delay could mean irreversible damage to other organs which would impact his transplant candidacy.

I encouraged him to obtain a second opinion (more on the importance of this later in the chapter). He researched his condition and saw an expert at another well-respected institution. She offered him the same assessment and recommendation and he agreed to transplant listing. I was relieved: I had provided the best information and options and he made an informed decision.

When the conversation ends in agreeing to disagree, don't think of this as a loss. End with respect. The patient-physician relationship, with the opportunity for future conversations, should endure.

9.6   The Patient Who Wants a Second Opinion

9.6.1   Encourage Second Opinions

They are never a bad thing, whether you are on the giving or receiving end. When a patient remains unconvinced by your recommended course of action, suggest a second opinion. Rather than a blow to your ego, a second opinion is a win–win situation. If the second opinion agrees with you, you will feel vindicated, and the patient will have renewed trust in you. If the second opinion does not agree with you, you may learn something, and the patient will have benefited from another perspective. By offering a second opinion to a patient, you and the patient will benefit no matter what the outcome. You will do your part to maintain mutual trust and respect and the patient-physician relationship stays strong.

Early in my career, a patient came to see me for evaluation of exertional angina refractory to medical management. A stress test was consistent with multivessel coronary artery disease, so I recommended an angiogram. I explained the indications, risks, alternatives, and benefits of an angiogram as well as potential outcomes. He was nervous and asked me to call his wife; I explained everything again to his wife on speaker phone. He remained unconvinced and though said he would call me to schedule the procedure, he never did.

A few weeks later, I received a courtesy call from another cardiologist: the patient had sought him out for a second opinion. The cardiologist agreed with my evaluation, scheduled the angiogram, and the patient was recovering from bypass surgery.

Looking back, I knew at the time that he was not confident in my recommendations despite my lengthy and patient explanations. I attempted to counter his reticence with more explanations which did not hit the mark. I'm grateful he sought out a second opinion though I realize I got lucky: what if he hadn't sought out another consultation and had a serious cardiac event?

Since then, when I have the sense that a patient is not buying what I'm selling, I consider the stakes. If they're high, like declining an angiogram to confirm multivessel coronary artery disease, I will preempt the patient by suggesting a second opinion and offer potential specialists who may be a good fit. Offer patients options when they need them most—you may save their life.

9.6.2 Learn from Being the Second Opinion

As the recipient of second opinions, I'm struck by the most common reason a patient seeks out a second opinion with me—and it's not my medical expertise. A patient with hypertension and high cholesterol came to see me for preoperative evaluation prior to back surgery. Another cardiologist had already evaluated him and performed a stress echocardiogram (though it was unnecessary as the patient had no symptoms with good exercise tolerance). Nonetheless, the stress test was normal as expected so there were no concerning cardiac issues warranting a second opinion. When I asked the patient why he sought out a second opinion, he explained that he was upset because the office nurse left him a message after the stress test: "You're fine." This bothered the patient. He wanted more than two words of reassurance on his voicemail.

The patient was the picture of health, and the normal stress test confirmed that. Still, I wasn't surprised that he came to see me—I have observed that lack of adequate communication is the most common reason that patients seek out second opinions. They have heard, from friends, family members, or other doctors, that I am good at listening and explaining. The lesson here: patients want to be heard and need to understand. If you listen and explain, they will be less likely to seek out second opinions.

When I review the notes of the physician who performed the initial evaluation, I almost always agree with their management. Second opinions rarely arise from concerns about medical decision-making. Rather, a patient-initiated second opinion is usually due to more mundane, non-medical issues like "the doctor didn't explain the test results to me" or "his office never called me back." These seemingly minor issues make the patient distrust the physician's medical competence. These second opinions are a constant reminder that effective communication is an essential component to optimal patient care.

9.7 Practicing the Art of Saying No

In the business world, the customer is always right. Does the same hold true in the world of healthcare? Are patients always right? Negative online reviews suggest the answer is yes: in anonymous online critiques, patients can vent about overpriced parking or unsmiling office staff, just as they would judge a restaurant or hair salon. If patients are customers and the customer is always right, is it the physician's job to always say yes?

I once walked into the examination room to see a new patient. When I asked what brought him to my office, he said, "I need you to order a coronary calcium scan." Stifling the urge to ask if he would also like his martini shaken or stirred, I took a deep breath and explained why my answer was no.

I'm accustomed to patients arriving to their appointments armed with a wish list. Sometimes, Dr. Google is accurate, and we achieve consensus. More often, the patient's investigation lacks context because they have no medical background, and it is impossible to be objective about one's own medical care. This applies to patients as well as doctors. As Sir William Osler said, "A physician who treats himself has a fool for a patient." In those situations, I work hard to convince the patient that what they think they want may not be what they need.

One could argue that, if a patient wants this scan or that pill, and I know the risks are minimal, why not acquiesce? At a high-end restaurant, if this patient ordered tartar sauce with his sole meunière, the waiter might shudder inwardly as they fulfilled his order. However, inappropriate medical testing puts patients at risk for more than a culinary *faux pas*. If there is a conflict between optimizing health and delivering satisfaction, choose the former at the expense of the latter. Even faced with the threat of an angry patient and a negative online review, do your best to convince the patient that a plan that promotes optimal health should confer the greatest satisfaction.

For a physician, saying no is harder than saying yes. Take comfort in knowing that a physician willing to take the risk to tell a patient want they need to hear, rather than what they want to hear, cares more about healing than pleasing. Strive to be this type of physician.

There is a misconception that more testing equates to better care, that a physician orders more tests because she knows more or cares more. At best, more testing may be simply the path of least resistance. At worst, more testing may give the illusion of better care. Just because something can be measured does not mean the measurement is medically relevant. For example, while some lipid particles are more likely to float and others are more likely to sink, will this information help a patient feel better or live longer? Unless there are very specific medical conditions, the answer is no.

If a waiter acquiesces to a cringe-worthy order for tartar sauce with sole meunière, the worst consequence might be indigestion. If a physician agrees to order a test that is not medically indicated, a patient could end up with an "incidentaloma," a finding of unclear significance that leads to further testing, anxiety, discomfort, and expense.

I cared for a patient who requested that his internist order a CT scan of the chest because his best friend was diagnosed with lung cancer. Unlike his best friend, the patient was young without risk factors so a CT scan was not medically indicated. This CT scan was a "fishing expedition" where the chance of an abnormal finding was so low that even if an abnormality were discovered, it was more likely to be a false-positive than a true-positive that could save a patient's life (Bayes' Theorem in action: your pre-test probability impacts your post-test probability). The risk of a false-positive finding: more unnecessary tests and risks of harm.

For this patient, the unnecessary CT scan revealed a lung nodule which led to a biopsy that confirmed that the nodule was nonspecific scar tissue. Perhaps this false alarm was a cause for celebration? Hard to celebrate when the biopsy was complicated by a pneumothorax requiring a 4-day hospital stay. Who can celebrate a normal result that should never have been investigated in the first place? For every unnecessary test that uncovers a rare life-saving diagnosis, many more lead to a cascade of more invasive and riskier testing that can cause harm.

What happened to the patient who requested a coronary calcium scan? A coronary calcium scan can provide an indication of possible future heart disease and can be helpful in deciding on whether a statin should be prescribed to reduce the risk of future cardiac events. He was already taking a statin with no side effects so the information from this scan would not impact his management. I was lucky: when I explained this, he realized that he was not missing out on important care. He agreed that it was best to avoiding unnecessary radiation and decided to forego the scan.

I might have been unlucky. He might have silently seethed and later posted an anonymous scathing review (more on these in Chap. 13). Remember, though, that you are not waiter in a nice restaurant, and you cannot adjust your practice to protect yourself from bad reviews. If the waiter declines your order for tartar sauce, you should write a negative review; the waiter has no right to judge your taste in food. Unlike a restaurant, a physician cannot prioritize satisfaction above all else; physicians are not waiters and patients are not customers. Medicine is not a service industry; it is a care industry. A request for medical testing should be based on more than a patient's desires; the downstream risks are greater than ruining a plate of fish.

Acquiescing to a test may result in instant gratification and a five-star review but long-term harm. Take the risk of instant dissatisfaction to protect the patient. Work to establish the trust it takes to convince the patient why declining to order a test is a sign of how much, rather than how little, you care. Share your medical reasoning. Follow your conscience, and practice the art of saying no.

9.8   Breaking Bad News

When I was a first-year medical student, a young man with leukemia spoke to our medical school class as part of the course on a patient's perspective on living with illness. He had experienced a few weeks of fatigue and then broke out in a rash which prompted him to present to a local emergency department. The rash was petechiae from thrombocytopenia and he was told he probably had leukemia. He described how he has given patient education pamphlets from the Leukemia and Lymphoma Society and told to call the oncology office on Monday morning for an appointment.

The story made an impression on me—I realized that there is no good way to receive bad news. No matter how well you deliver it, the patient will hear very little of what you say, and they will always associate you with the bad news. However, there are strategies you can employ to make the delivery as effective and compassionate as possible, though it will never be pleasant.

9.8.1   Step 1: Have a Concrete Action Plan

One of the most awful feelings in medicine is the state of limbo where you know the bad news and the patient does not (yet). As a fellow, I cared for a patient who had advanced heart failure requiring heart transplantation. He was the perfect patient, an engineer who kept meticulous track of his medications and vital signs and even corrected spelling errors in the heart transplant orientation manual (it had not been edited in years and no one else had read it so carefully).

I knew he would be the perfect transplant candidate until a routine screening chest CT scan uncovered the worst unanticipated finding: a mass suspicious for lung cancer. He had dozens of prior chest x-rays and the mass had not been apparent. As bad luck would have it, the mass was in the left upper chest, masked by his implantable defibrillator. When I clicked open the chest CT report, my heart sank. He would never be a candidate for heart transplantation, and it would be a race to the death: advanced heart failure or lung cancer. I knew that it should be me, not my attending physician, to break the news to him.

I was inexperienced. I needed a plan and didn't have one; I didn't know what to say. My mentor gave me the best advice: don't just drop the bomb, start the clean-up. The bad news is the bomb; the next steps are the clean-up. My mentor walked me through the discussion: after I delivered the bad news, after the patient absorbed it, he would want to know what happens next. I needed to do the groundwork to provide him with the answers.

So, before I reached out to the patient, I called my favorite oncologist. If he were to see my patient in consultation, what would the next steps be? He explained that he would order a PET scan and refer the patient to a thoracic surgeon for resection. I scheduled an appointment for the patient with the oncologist and felt a little better. While the bomb would cause devastating damage, at least I had a plan to salvage whatever possible from the wreckage.

9.8.2 Step 2: Determine the Delivery

Despite having a plan in place, I was still unsure about how to deliver the bad news. His next appointment wasn't for a week, and I didn't want him to wait that long. Should I give the bad news over the phone? Should I ask him to move up his appointment? Which was worse, hearing the news over the phone, or receiving a call to move up his appointment without knowing why?

My mentor again came to the rescue. Of course, for an experienced clinician, situations like this happen all the time. She advised me to tailor my approach to the patient. Knowing the patient as I did, what would be worse: fretting about an upcoming appointment, knowing he was driving, parking, checking in to hear bad news, or receiving it sooner over the phone? In the end, I knew this patient would prefer the latter. I called him, asked him if he could put his wife on speaker phone, and broke the news.

Years ago, video visits were not an option as they are now. Still, relaying bad news remotely, whether over video or phone, can be challenging. In both cases, you cannot offer the same direct comfort as during an in-person visit. If this happened today, would I choose video over phone? It depends on the patient. For some less technologically adept patients, the video connection is challenging compared to the ease of a phone call. My mentor's advice still rings true: tailor the approach to the patient.

9.8.3 Step 3: Let the News Register

Of course, it was horrible to deliver the terrible news. I explained the medical facts clearly and offered the patient and his wife an honest differential diagnosis: "The CT scan of your chest showed a mass in your lung. That mass is probably cancer. I know this is horrible news. I want to talk about what this means." We did not yet know if the mass was cancer, but I purposely used the "C" word based on my mentor's advice. When you deliver bad news, patients will immediately go to the worst-case scenario. It might seem that avoiding the elephant in the room, offering the most positive spin, provides the most comfort. Actually, that approach provides more comfort to you, not to the patient. Have the courage to voice the patient's greatest fears so you can make a plan to address them.

I knew that even though I kept talking after dropping the bomb of the diagnosis, they wouldn't hear what I was saying. Instead of launching into the plan, I repeated the facts and their anticipated questions: "I know it must seem strange that there could be a mass that's probably lung cancer when you've never smoked. It wasn't picked up on chest x-ray because the defibrillator inadvertently hid the mass. It's not surprising that you haven't had symptoms. Sometimes these masses don't cause symptoms. It's also possible that some of your heart failure symptoms, the fatigue, weight loss, cough, were from the mass too." This interlude, for reiterating and anticipating questions, allows the patient time and space to process and ask more questions.

9.8.4 Step 4: Explain the Plan

After explaining the medical facts, the next step is to move on to the plan for diagnosis, treatment, and prognosis. I like to say, "The next steps are to figure out what this is, what you need to do about it, and what it means for your life moving forward. Here is our plan to get the process started."

In this specific situation, I told the patient and his wife: "I'm not an oncologist, so I can't tell you exactly what this is, though I spoke with an oncologist before calling you and he agrees that it is likely cancer. The next steps would be to see him, have a PET scan to assess for possible spread, and meet with a thoracic surgeon to talk about surgical resection. I've set up the appointment with the oncologist—can I give you the date/time?" Sometimes patients aren't ready for the next steps yet, and still want to absorb the facts. Other patients go into planning mode immediately. Either way, let the patient guide the pace of the discussion.

9.8.5 Step 5: Make the Promise

The final step is to make a promise. You cannot make a promise that everything will be okay, but you can promise to always be there. What I say to patients is: "I know we have more questions than answers; I promise to always have a plan to get the answers. I will always be honest with you, whether the news is good or bad." Remember: honesty and humility are the ethos of an experienced physician.

9.8.6 Step 6: Circle Back

In a day or two, call the patient back to see how the news is settling, to ensure the follow up plan is in place, and to answer additional questions. Patients will go through the stages of grieving when they receive terrible news: denial, anger, bargaining, grief, and acceptance. The stages can happen in any order and last as long as they need to. Meet the patient where they are as you help them through the process.

My patient's story, as expected, did not have a happy ending. I saw him regularly during his cancer treatments, though there was little I could do except peel away guideline-directed medical therapy as his hypotension and renal dysfunction worsened. One of the last times I saw him, his wife was pushing his wheelchair into an elevator. She had aged years in just a few months and he was slumped, jaundiced with vacant eyes. I held the elevator door and smiled as I tried to hide my shock.

She tried to smile too and thanked me for continuing to be his doctor even though he was no longer a transplant candidate. I felt both shame and grief; while I had not caused the cancer, I had set them down this path of suffering and could not fix him. I had imagined how wonderful his life would be after heart transplantation: joking with him in clinic, hearing stories about his volunteer work in the hospital helping other transplant candidates with the process, revising the patient orientation manual together. I had not imagined his current state.

I did not share my sorrow; what was the point? She had enough grief of her own, which I would have gladly absorbed for the duration of our elevator ride. Amazingly, she showed me only grace and gratitude. I was humbled and this interaction was a revelation: being present can be enough. Sustain and maintain the patient-physician relationship even when cure of the patient's disease is no longer possible.

To sum up, when it comes to giving bad news, think of it in 5 steps:

(1) Preparation: especially when you have uncovered a bad finding that is not in your area of expertise, reach out to a trusted colleague for advice on the next steps to determine the diagnosis, treatment, and prognosis.
(2) The honest differential diagnosis: when you tell patients about an awful test result, they will immediately fear the worst, and the worst is often cancer. Call out the elephant in the room. I will say: "The best-case scenario is that it is X, and the worst-case scenario is that it is Y. My experience and consultation with colleagues with expertise in this area tell me that it's most likely Z."
(3) The plan: Delivering bad news is awful. You are dividing a patient's life into the before, when everything was okay, to after, when everything changed for the worst. You cannot make it better, but you can make it easier to understand. Delivering bad news without a plan is cruel. Don't just drop the bomb; arrange the clean-up. Delivering bad news with a plan give patients something constructive to focus on.
(4) The reiteration: Much of what you say will be lost to the roar of the adrenaline surge in their head. Whenever possible, break the news with a loved one there as a second set of eyes and ears. Also, repeat yourself until it appears that they have understood.
(5) The promise: I want patients to know that I will be honest and will not abandon them. That's why I always promise that even if we don't have all the answers, we'll make a plan to get them.
(6) Circle back: Meet the patient where they are in the stages of grief as they process the terrible news and move towards acceptance.

9.9 When You don't Know

The two hallmarks of an experienced physician are honesty and humility. There are good ways to say,"I don't know", and not-so-good ways. "I don't know" is never the end of a conversation. Whether you're speaking with your colleagues, attending physicians, or patients, honesty is important, and honesty combined with initiative is essential.

9.9.1 Honesty on Rounds

Consider these scenarios:

The scene: morning rounds.

Attending physician: What about the CT scan we discussed on rounds yesterday?

Trainee 1: I believe it was ordered.

Trainee 2: I'm not sure if it was ordered.

Trainee 3: I don't know if it was ordered. I forgot to check but I'll check now.

Trainee 1 decided to hedge. To the trained ear of an attending physician, a hedged answer is a non-answer. A hedged answer indicates the speaker is more interested in covering up for potential errors than caring for patients. Don't hedge.

Trainee 2 also decided to hedge though they edged closer to the truth. Still, what is supposed to happen next? It's not enough to admit that you dropped the ball; you need to pick the ball back up. "I don't know" may start the discussion, but it will not end it.

Trainee 3 was honest and had a plan. The attending physician may be chagrined that the trainee forgot an essential component of patient care. However, the attending would also have respect for a trainee who identified the error and sought to rectify it.

9.9.2 Honesty with Patients

When a patient asks you a question, and you don't know the answer, what should you do?

Sometimes, there is no clear answer. If a patient asks how long their heart transplant surgery will take, there are many reasons for me to honestly tell them I don't know. First, I'm not a surgeon, so I have little conception of what transpires during surgery. Second, no one can predict the range of factors which impact the duration of the surgery. Third, the patient is not just interested in how long they'll be in the operating room; it's important to address the emotion behind the question.

The stepwise approach to saying "I don't know" to a patient is: honesty, direct the patient to the right source, refocus the priorities for their care, and address the emotion behind the question.

One approach to respond to this question: "I'm not a heart transplant surgeon, so I can't say for sure how long the surgery will last [*honesty*]. You'll be seeing the surgeon later this morning and they can give you a better idea [*direct the patient to the right source*]."

What about the emotion behind the question? A patient who asks about the duration of the transplant operation may really be asking about the risks and their chances of survival. If you sense fear behind the question, address it: "The surgery takes as long as it needs to take [*refocus the priorities*]. If you were too high risk to undergo heart transplantation, we would not be discussing it. All surgery has risks, but your odds of having a healthy life are better with a transplant than without [*address the emotion behind the question*]."

There are also ways to avoid having to say "I don't know" when you should know—preparation. If a patient with cardiomyopathy associated with muscular dystrophy is scheduled to see me, I will read up in advance and have a concrete action plan (with references) in my notes. I'm less familiar with the cardiac surveillance strategies for different forms of muscular dystrophy and this approach allows me to ensure that I have done the necessary research to provide optimal patient care. Reason #734 why reviewing records in advance of a patient's appointment is essential: you will be comfortable managing even less familiar conditions and you will not have to say, "I don't know."

9.9.3   End-of-Life Care

I was once rounding in the intensive care unit on (yet another) patient with atrial fibrillation with rapid ventricular response. As I was exiting the ICU, I encountered a disturbing sight: another patient of mine, whom I had evaluated months prior to assess his cardiac candidacy for liver transplantation, was in cardiac arrest.

A nurse was performing chest compressions, an anesthesiologist was preparing to intubate, and the senior resident was directing the code. Outside the room, the patient's wife and daughter stood in shock as the liver transplant surgery fellow explained the situation.

I knew this fellow well and had great respect for his clinical judgment and work ethic (does anyone work harder than a liver transplant surgery fellow?). Still, I was aghast when I overheard his conversation with the family. It went along the lines of, "His heart has stopped, and we are coding him. Do you want us to do everything?".

Even though I hadn't seen the patient in months, I couldn't stand by as the fellow broke one of the cardinal rules of end-of-life care: family members never make medical decisions. I stepped closer, reintroduced myself, and took over. The fellow was not upset; rather, he was surprised and relieved. Together, we explained the medical situation to the family.

The fellow described the Candida fungemia, renal failure, and adult respiratory distress syndrome that had culminated in post-transplant liver failure and now a cardiac arrest. I explained that even if the patient survived the cardiac arrest, his other organs were too severely injured to allow for meaningful recovery. The medical situation was clear and the explanation, while devastating, was honest. Resuscitative efforts were futile in this situation and the family grasped the terrible news that there was no hope and that they were not in control of his fate.

The patient did not survive, which was a tragedy. The family was not made to feel responsible for the decision of whether he lived or died, which would have been a greater tragedy still. The fellow thanked me for my help. He understood the medical reality though sharing it honestly made him uncomfortable. He did not want to be cruel and rob the family of their hope for the best outcome. I advised him that it was even crueler to give false hope. As physicians, delivering bad news is our duty. I like to think that this experience gave him courage to face future family discussions with honesty and compassion.

When I consider end-of-life situations, certain rules come to mind.

9.9.4 Step 1: Know All the Facts; Use Only the Ones the Families Need to Hear

When you are discussing end-of-life situations with families, always be more prepared with the medical facts than you need to be and let the family guide you regarding how much detail to provide. Prepare in advance and have brief notes: dates of admissions and decompensations, the status of every organ system, the identity of each infectious organism and the antimicrobials used to treat them, the names and plans of all the involved consultants, and so on. If needed, make your consultants work for you: prod them to provide the specific prognosis related to their organ system. Consider an invitation to be present at the family meeting if their organ system is the major driver of prognosis and outside your sphere of expertise.

When you meet with the family, start with a general overview of the hospitalization: where it began and how the patient has progressed. Families will let you know how much they want to know. Some families will listen and allow you to lead the discussion. Others will inquire about details big and small. Why do some families need to know everything? They may feel that knowledge is power and if they understand the situation, they can control the outcome. They may also want to assess your fund of knowledge as a marker of your competence. In any case, preparation will again inspire the trust essential for providing optimal patient care.

9.9.5 Step 2: Frame Best-Case and Worst-Case Scenarios

After going through the patient's trajectory by organ system, move on to best- and worst-case scenarios (aided, as needed, with input from the consultants). Sometimes, even the best-case scenario is not that great, and involves months in the hospital followed by rehabilitation or skilled nursing facility with little hope of independent life. Paint this picture as clearly and specifically as possible. Use words like "die" and "death" rather than euphemisms like "pass away." Describe, to the best of your medical knowledge, what life will look like: will the patient be able to care for themselves, engage in hobbies they enjoyed, interact with their loved ones? Let the family know that while you never want to give bad news, you will always be honest. You will never hide the truth to spare their feelings.

9.9.6   Step 3. Explore the patient's Goals, Values, and Preferences

Often, I have end-of-life discussions with patients and families that I have known for years. In these cases, the patient and their family trust my medical decision-making and my understanding of the patient's goals, values, and preferences. Even if you don't know the patient or their family well, this trust can be forged quickly with the above steps and by learning what you can about the patient.

If I know the patient well, I will say, "Knowing him as I do, here is what I think he would have wanted. What do you think?" If I have just met the patient, I'll ask the family to tell me about him: what he enjoyed, what he valued. I will say, "Hearing about what was important to him, my sense is this may be the right medical path. Tell me what you think."

It can also be helpful to frame possible options for patients and families, to model decision-making. You can say, "Some patients, when faced with this prognosis, feel the quality of life they would achieve is not acceptable. They choose to let nature take its course without further attempts to reverse the condition. In this case, I talk to patients about what dying might look like. Other patients feel differently: exhausting all options is important to them, and they want to push forward until there is no hope of recovery. There is no right answer in this situation, and your preferences may change as times goes on—but what seems right to you now?".

9.9.7   Step 4. Make the Promise

Offer an explicit promise: you will never ask the patient nor their family to make medical decisions. Families should never feel like they are "pulling the plug" because they are not. Rather, you will explain the medical facts. You will offer a medical recommendation based on the medical facts. If there are decisions that depend on the patient's goals, values, and preferences, you will explain those branch points and options.

Don't allow a discussion about "code status" to break this promise to the patient and their family: patients and families never make medical decisions. Code status is not a menu and should not be presented as such: do you want CPR, intubation, medications to jump start your heart? A laundry list like this is medically inappropriate and puts patients and families in the untenable position of a medical decision-maker. If CPR or intubation is not appropriate given their medical condition, say so: "You are very sick. If the worst were to happen, and your heart were to stop beating or you were to stop breathing, this would be a sign that your body has given up. Attempts to restart your heart with chest compressions or place a breathing tube would result in more suffering. These measures would not save your life or achieve the quality of life that is important to you. My medical recommendation is that we do not perform CPR or intubation if it comes to that. Tell me what you think about my recommendation."

9.9.8   Step 5. Come to Consensus

The patient and their family may agree or disagree with your medical recommendations on end-of-life care. That's okay—as with every decision in medicine, shared decision-making, considering the patient's goals, values, and preferences, is essential. However, this consensus-building process still requires your medical decision. Shared decision-making is not abdication of medical decision-making. Shared decision-making starts with your medical recommendation, incorporates the patient's wishes, and ends with a concrete action plan.

9.10   More Thoughts About End-of-Life Care

9.10.1   There Should be Grief

It is awful to watch a patient or family members grieve—though it is necessary. In the throes of an end-of-life discussion, if there is no grief, then you have not done your job. Tears often mean that you have been heard and understood. I once had to counsel a family that their beloved son had suffered a massive stroke after heart surgery and would never wake up. We had daily family meetings where I explained his unresponsive state and the inexorable subsequent breakdown of his body with infection and organ failure. In the face of grim medical facts, his parents remained steadfast in their hope for a miracle.

Then one day, a week into his hospitalization, I had to break more bad news: his leg, ischemic from a vascular access injury, was now gangrenous. On hearing this, his mother started to cry. Neither the stroke, nor the sepsis, renal failure, small bowel obstruction, or adult respiratory distress syndrome bothered her. She finally realized how sick he was, and that he would not recover, when she learned that he would lose his leg. She said that her son, a track star in high school, would never want to live without a leg.

As she cried, and her husband fought back tears, it was clear that they finally accepted the horrible truth: he would never again be the young man whom they adored. Watching a family dissolve as they lose the last bit of hope is gut-wrenching. Still, there is a measure of relief. You have guided them through the worst time in their lives to the point of acceptance. Acceptance is the goal. Once the family focuses their energy on accepting the tragic prognosis instead of trying to fight it, the healing process can begin.

9.10.2   *You Do not Have a Crystal Ball*

If the family is at peace with cessation of life-prolonging measures and wants to know how long until their loved one dies, rest assured that your prediction will rarely be correct. If you say a day, it will be a week and if you say a week, it will be a day. Either way, the family will either live in a perpetual state of grief waiting for the worst that takes too long to come or else they will be caught off guard because it happens sooner than you said. In most cases, I make sure to emphasize that death happens on its own timeline: hours to days to weeks, and the body knows best.

9.10.3   *Your Right Answer May Not Be Their Right Answer*

Who is to say what is a good death? The bone marrow transplant service horrified me as an intern. Patients arrived appearing relatively healthy and within days were ravaged by weakness and pallor and mouth sores and hair loss. Witnessing the devastation, I asked my attending if he would ever have a bone marrow transplant himself. He said that before he had children, he would have said no. After he became a father, he realized that he would endure any suffering if it offered the chance of more time with his kids. Unmarried and childless at the time, I was skeptical; decades later, his words ring true. Our goals, values, and preferences factor into our definition of a good death.

I cared for a heart transplant recipient with breast cancer which had spread to her lungs. She was in respiratory failure and ventilator dependent. She had been my patient for about a decade when she became ill and ultimately ended up in the intensive care unit with a tracheostomy, alert yet unable to speak, and stuck in a limbo of too healthy to die (every organ save her lungs worked properly) and too sick to live (her cancer was too advanced to benefit from chemotherapy).

We explained to her and her mother, an ever-present fixture at her bedside, that she would die in the hospital. We were just waiting for the inevitable, a race to the death that could take weeks or months, the leading contenders of her demise being sepsis or brain metastases. Still, she would not give up. Every day, with a portable ventilator, she walked laps around the ICU, her mother cheering her on. Every day, I felt terrible because we were not curing her and I knew we never would; we were delaying the inevitable, treading water, waiting for something bad to happen.

Eventually, it did: she developed brain metastases. Once she was no longer conscious, her mother accepted her fate and let her daughter go. Perhaps the process took a few weeks longer than it should have, medically. Perhaps we spent countless thousands of healthcare dollars on her that could have been better spent on childhood vaccinations in underdeveloped countries.

We were frustrated because the patient and her mother would not believe us when we shared her grim prognosis. They came to terms with her prognosis on their own timeline. If we had coerced the patient or her mother to stop life-sustaining measures before they were ready, we would have saved ourselves weeks of frustration. We would have saved ourselves those weeks, however, at the expense of her mother's guilt which would have lasted a lifetime. The trade-off, our weeks of frustration, for her mother's years of peace, was worth it to us.

You don't just treat the patient in end-of-life care, you treat the family as well. When you treat the family, the pain or inconvenience or medical inelegance of their death may stay with you for a few days, or a few weeks, but that death will stay with the family forever. Do your best to remove guilt from the equation: family members should never feel as if they are steering the medical course. When possible, you should allow them to chart the course that aligns with their goals, values, and preferences. All suffering is not created equal, and sometimes the suffering of giving up is worse than the many indignities of chronic ICU care.

The patient died on her own terms with dignity and pride. She did not suffer; she spent her final days fighting and that mattered to her. I'm still not sure if we, as the medical team, made the right decision for the hospital or society at large; despite the seemingly limitless resources of a big-city hospital, there were likely other patients who could have occupied this bed and lived. While we were expending resources on a patient who would never survive, were there patients who did not receive life-saving care? Still, I think of her at the end, nodding and giving me a thumbs up as she pulled the portable ventilator down the hallway of the intensive care unit, mother strong by her side. I have not kept in touch with her mother though I suspect that even now, years later, she grieves her daughter's death. I can only hope that she is at peace because her daughter died on her own terms. When I think of this patient, and her mother, I'd like to believe we did the best we could– for them both.

9.11   Final Thoughts

The tough conversations are challenging because the stakes are high. Work with your patient so they understand that your only priority is their health. Incorporate the patient's goals, values, and preferences with your medical recommendations to make a concrete action plan. Accept that you cannot please or convince everyone. Do your best to preserve the patient-physician relationship because the end of the conversation is not the end of the relationship.

Reference

Singh Ospina N, Phillips KA, Rodriguez-Gutierrez R, Castaneda-Guarderas A, Gionfriddo MR, Branda ME, Montori VM. Eliciting the patient's agenda-secondary analysis of recorded clinical encounters. J Gen Intern Med. 2019;34:36–40.

Part IV
Optimizing the Care of Patients and Yourself

Chapter 10
The Patient-Physician Bond

The best, and worst, aspect of medicine for me is chronic care. Some physicians are drawn to the shift work of hospitalist or emergency medicine because it eschews the long-term relationships that blur the boundaries between one's personal and professional lives. It's easier to leave work behind when someone, interchangeable with you, is now caring for the patients. It's harder to leave work behind when you know that your presence, over that of any other physician of comparable skill and expertise, will bring the patient and their family comfort in difficult times.

When a patient wants you and only you, the responsibility can be exasperating, gratifying, and humbling. I cared for a young man who presented with cardiogenic shock from presumed viral myocarditis. One day, he was a handsome college athlete, golden child of his fraternity, and the next he was on extracorporeal membrane life support awaiting a heart transplant. He did very well, of course, because youth afforded him resilience and he was back on campus, golden child once more, within months. Then a routine biopsy just before Thanksgiving showed rejection. It was mild and would require only an increase in oral corticosteroids with a follow-up biopsy a few weeks later. Still, when the heart transplant nurse coordinator called to deliver the news on the Wednesday before Thanksgiving, he was distraught.

I was on vacation and blissfully unaware, deep in the midst of my annual Thanksgiving preparations, complete with a grocery list spreadsheet and a timeline that started the Sunday before Thanksgiving and ended, in 30-min increments, at noon on the big day. On Thanksgiving morning, while checking a recipe on my phone, I noticed an alert from the hospital's electronic medical records app.

The alert was a message from the nurse coordinator. Though she had reassured the patient that the biopsy findings were not dangerous, he was inconsolable and wanted to speak to me. The coordinator explained that I was on vacation and offered to have another physician call him. Nonetheless, he begged her to reach out to me, and she sent me the message which I found on Thanksgiving morning.

My first instinct was mild irritation. The medical aspect of his care was perfect: an appropriately timed routine biopsy uncovered an unanticipated, though not unexpected finding, and the correct treatment plan had been implemented. My input would

M. Kittleson, *Mastering the Art of Patient Care*,
https://doi.org/10.1007/978-3-031-20920-8_10

not impact the outcome. My second instinct was guilt. Just a year prior, his parents had experienced a very different Thanksgiving, never imagining their healthy son would soon be in the intensive care unit straddling the line between life and death. I had focused on the importance of medical management and ignored the other essential half of optimal patient care: communication and connection.

My patient and his parents had gamely adapted to their new world of medications and doctor visits and blood draws and biopsies. When they finally took a proverbial deep breath and let themselves plan for his future once again, they were blindsided by a biopsy showing rejection. They were faced with the realization that something awful could still happen when they least expected. They did not need my medical knowledge. They needed my reassurance and of course I would provide that while on vacation on Thanksgiving morning.

I called. His mom tripped over her words in gratitude and woke her son just to talk to me. Just my voice, reiterating the exact same message as the nurse coordinator, was enough. I put the Thanksgiving sides in the oven to rewarm, tented foil over the resting turkey, and threw away the completed spreadsheet. Though I busied myself with these Thanksgiving tasks, I could not escape my shame and discomfort. I was ashamed of my knee-jerk irritation and uncomfortable with the family's faith in me. I knew that my words had no magical power. Just because I told them that the biopsy was no cause for concern was no guarantee that he would not have more serious issues down the line.

Still, the irritation and discomfort faded and were replaced by gratitude. It was an honor to have such a relationship, with hundreds of patients and their families, borne of years of care though times of celebration and mourning. A simple phone call was all it took and, in the end, we both had a nice Thanksgiving.

Accept the moments of irritation, guilt, and discomfort along with those of joy and gratitude. How extraordinary, to be the one special doctor for a patient and their family. This bond may seem at times burdensome, yet it is a gift. As you cross the bridge from inexperience to experience, you will appreciate these special moments. The knee-jerk irritation will diminish, replaced by gratitude, as your empathy grows.

There are ways to forge effective connections with your patients to strengthen the patient-physician bond. Here are some tips, built on experience, to build a relationship of mutual trust and respect.

10.1   Addressing Patients

10.1.1   Introductions

I am old-fashioned. I start by calling all patients Mr., Ms., or Dr. unless they invite me to use their first name. Err on the side of formality until the patient gives you permission to be less formal. Admittedly, I have relaxed this rule as I've aged: it feels ridiculous to address a patient young enough to be my kid as Mr. or Ms.—and I'll say, "Since I'm older than you, I'm going to call you by your first name!".

Get in the habit of asking patients, when you first meet them, how to pronounce their names. I once cared for a patient in the hospital whom I had known for years. When I entered the room with my team on rounds and introduced him, he corrected my pronunciation. He said, "Doc, I love you, but that's not actually how you pronounce my name." It turns out that I had been placing the emphasis on the first instead of second syllable for all the years I'd known him. I am not sure why he never corrected me sooner; perhaps he considered this an opportunity to finally set the record straight. The timing, while curious, did afford me an opportunity to provide my trainees with a teaching point: unless entirely obvious, always ask if you're pronouncing someone's name correctly. This way, you can avoid embarrassing confrontations in front of your team years later. It's okay to ask for a reminder if you forget after the first introduction; patients will appreciate your concern and attention to detail.

When meeting patients, never presume to know who is with them: always ask. Having mistaken fathers for husbands and daughters for wives, I can tell you that foot-mouth extraction is painful and rarely 100% successful. The best approach, "Who is this with you today?".

10.1.2 Patients with Dementia or Learning Disabilities

Sometimes patients cannot communicate due to dementia or learning disabilities. In medical school, I observed how one attending physician evaluated a patient with dementia. He sat by the side of her bed, looked her in the eye, and asked questions. Sometimes she answered and sometimes her sister, ever present at the bedside, chimed in. He obtained all the necessary information from the patient and her sister and as we left the room, the patient's sister thanked him. She appreciated my attending's patience because so many clinicians spoke only to her and not to the patient. By addressing the patient directly, my attending showed that he cared about the patient as a person, not just as a collection of diagnoses.

Thanks to this fleeting mentor on a 2-week internal medicine rotation, I try to always address the patient directly, giving them the benefit of the doubt and preserving their dignity. They will either (1) understand and respond appropriately; (2) understand and not respond appropriately and a caregiver will interject and explain; or (3) not understand and not respond, allowing the caregiver to chime in. Regardless, it's a win–win situation: you have allowed the patient to maintain their dignity and autonomy, you have shown the caregiver that you value the patient as a person, and you have obtained the needed information. The loved ones of patients with dementia particularly appreciate the effort. They remember who the patient was before dementia; they are grateful that you understand that there is a person somewhere inside the diminishing illness.

10.1.3   Unresponsive Patients

What about patients who are sedated or unresponsive? I have cared for many patients in the intensive care unit who are intubated and sedated. It's striking to hear the ICU experiences of those who recover: the pain, loud noises, snatches of gentle words or music. I once saw a patient for the first time in clinic. When I introduced myself, he said, "I recognize your voice. I know we've met before!" In fact, we had, months earlier in the ICU when he was intubated and sedated. Though we had never had a conversation, I had introduced myself every morning on rounds as I examined him and that must have penetrated his consciousness. This encounter reinforced the importance of talking to patients no matter what their apparent level of consciousness. It was the first time he spoke to me, yet we already had a connection.

Because I can never be sure what a sedated or unconscious patient will absorb, I address them directly when I'm examining them or doing procedures like placement of central venous access. This is helpful for many reasons: (1) you can't be sure what they comprehend and addressing them directly may reduce fear and confusion; and (2) it reminds you that they are a person and not a collection of diagnoses; and (3) it keeps you in the habit of always narrating your actions for patients.

10.2   Managing Expectations

As with most things in life, it is important to manage expectations. What's the best way to manage expectations? Underpromise and overdeliver. Appropriately tempering a patient's expectations will help them deal with the frustrations of being a patient. Some frustrations are avoidable and others are not. Managing expectations means you will help patients distinguish poor service, which may be out of your control, from poor care, which is not.

10.2.1   Hospital Standard Time

Anyone who has spent too much time in a medical setting, whether as a physician, patient, or caregiver, knows that tests or interventions rarely happen on time. When a patient is scared, sleep-deprived, and hungry, the uncertainty can be overwhelming. In these situations, I explain "hospital standard time."

If the patient is scheduled for an angiogram at 10 am, the angiogram may not happen until 4 pm, because emergencies can interrupt the lineup of scheduled procedures and some cases take longer than expected. To put things in perspective, remind the patient that it's wonderful to not be the emergency. Emphasize that cases may run long because the physicians will spend as much time as needed on every patient—including them.

Explaining hospital standard time serves two purposes: managing expectations and reframing them. The goal in the hospital is not to have everything done on time (though that would be nice for all involved). Rather, the goal is to have everything done safely and successfully—and safety and success takes precedence over punctuality. It's not that the patient doesn't know this; when patients are nervous and afraid, everything seems worse. Do your part to explain the priorities of their care to make things better.

10.2.2 Discharge Planning

If a patient is admitted to the hospital with heart failure, and you tell the patient they'll stay 3 days and they end up staying 5 days, they're disappointed. If you tell the patient they'll stay 7 days and they stay 5 days, you're a miracle worker. Same reality, different expectations. Manage expectations around discharge planning and better yet, provide criteria for discharge instead of days. Rather than telling the patient that they'll probably be in the hospital for 3–4 more days, tell them that they'll be in the hospital until certain criteria are met: walking around free of pain, eating a regular diet, with normal laboratories values, or whatever the case dictates.

Remind them that their body will know when it's time. Shift the focus of discharge from you ("my doctor won't let me leave the hospital!") to them ("my body needs to accomplish these tasks before I'm ready to leave!"). The patient controls so little in the hospital. When they actually have the opportunity to be in control, empower them. Focus their effort where it counts.

The day of discharge should never be a surprise to the patient. Disposition is a plant that you have to water for it to bloom. Ensure that the patient has a place to go, a way to get there, and is strong enough to be there with the support available. If you do not ensure these essential components are in place, you will be faced with a patient who may be medically ready to leave the hospital but has no home, no ride, or inadequate strength to care for themselves at home.

Finally, be clear about who's making the discharge decisions, especially if it's not you. If you're the consultant and the patient asks when they'll be discharged, it's not up to you to say. Let them know that the issue for which you are consulting is resolved, which is great news, and that the primary team will discuss the timing of discharge. Managing expectations means that you will defer and direct the patient to the appropriate decision-maker when necessary.

10.2.3 Side Effects

Prepare patients for side effects and explain which side effects are dangerous and which are not. Balance the importance of the medication with the tolerability of the side effect. I will tell patients that ACE inhibitors may cause a cough and nondihydropyridine calcium channel blockers may cause edema: I emphasize that neither side effect is dangerous and if tolerable, the important medication can be continued.

10.2.4 The Results of Tests/Interventions

As noted in Chap. 5, when you send a patient for a test, explain why you're ordering it, the possible results, and the plan for each result. For example, if the patient is scheduled for a stress test to diagnose the source of chest pain, let the patient know that the stress test may be (1) positive, suggestive of coronary artery disease, negative; (2) negative, suggestive of no coronary artery disease; or (3) indeterminate, where the results are not accurate, and more testing may be needed. Explain that a positive stress test may require adjustment in medications or an angiogram depending on the degree of abnormality.

If a patient with exertional chest discomfort and abnormal stress test undergoes an angiogram, explain that the angiogram may show: (1) blockages for which stents will be placed; (2) significant disease best fixed with bypass surgery; (3) minor or diffuse blockages not amenable to revascularization and requiring medical optimization; or (4) no blockages, which may mean that the chest pain is not cardiac in origin and the stress test is wrong, or that there is a rarer cardiac cause that warrants further investigation.

When the range of possibilities is explained, the patient is prepared for what may come next and is not surprised, disappointed, or upset by an unexpected finding. This is important for the patient and forces you to have a plan for a positive, negative, and indeterminate result. And if you don't have a plan, or if the results don't change the plan, then think twice about ordering the test.

10.3 Care Versus Service

It is our job to demonstrate to patients that outstanding care is essential and good service is not. Remember the old aphorism discussed in Chap. 6: patients want three things: availability, affability, and ability (in that order). What happens when availability and affability (service) trump ability (care)? I worked in a hospital where there was a unit with shiny wood laminate floors and afternoon tea reserved for very important people. When a patient went into cardiac arrest, no one could find the bag-valve-mask for precious minutes; it was hidden behind fancy wood paneling. I'm sure the patient satisfaction scores on that unit were very high, though one could argue that the most important question on such a survey should be, "Did you live, or did you die?".

10.3.1 Delays Are the Luxury of the Healthy

One lesson I learned as a patient: it's OK to wait your turn (see *Hospital Standard Time*, above). I've told you that I've called the pediatrician's answering service late at night about a fevering toddler. I felt the irrational parental fear, the frustration with the endless automated phone tree, the grating hold music, and interminable wait for the pediatrician to call back. Still, I know that just because I want an immediate response doesn't mean that, medically, I need that immediate response.

In fact, I yearned for the frustrating delays of the pediatrician's on-call phone tree when my son contracted RSV pneumonia. The controlled chaos that ensued after he was noted to be hypoxemic in urgent care, from initiation of supplemental oxygen to chest x-ray to placement of the intravenous line to the ambulance ride to a nearby hospital was medically necessary—and overwhelming. I wanted to be the mom of a healthy 4-year-old, frustrated with delays, rather than the mom of a son sick enough to inspire the whirlwind of a medical emergency.

When I keep a patient waiting, I apologize and make a joke to illustrate the difference between poor care and poor service: I tell patients the delay wasn't because I was drinking coffee or watching television. Explain that waiting is the luxury of the healthy. Promise the patient that you will give them all the time they need, even if it means that you're late for the patients scheduled after them.

10.3.2 Trust the Experts

Another lesson I learned as a patient: trust the experts. I chose my obstetrician because he was experienced. When I was admitted to the hospital in labor and asked about my birth plan, I said, "My birth plan is Dr. B." (And an epidural, let's be honest).

The music and the lights and the decision to ingest the placenta were window dressing. All I needed was a healthy baby, and Dr. B was my best shot to make that happen. I wish patients knew that Dr. Google is not a substitute for years of training and practice. Reading something on a "medical" website is not the same as understanding the context and limitations of the information. Judgment and experience cannot be intuited from a webpage.

How can you convince patients of this? First, you'll demonstrate your competence through preparation. Second, you'll be direct and honest about your expertise. When a patient asks for antibiotics for a viral upper respiratory infection or a stress test to evaluate noncardiac chest pain, don't be afraid to explain that you know more than they do and point out the flaws in their reasoning (more on Practicing the Art of Saying No in Chap. 12). You can be direct, honest, and still preserve the patient-physician bond.

10.3.3 Know When to Expedite

By the same token, as discussed in Chap. 6, it's important to recognize when better service does mean better care. A heart transplant patient saw me for a routine follow-up visit. He had a lung nodule incidentally noted on chest X-ray and was scheduled to see a pulmonologist two weeks later. In addition to the lung nodule, he had a 20-lb unintentional weight loss, undoubtedly the most concerning associated symptom indicating a serious underlying diagnosis.

I did not want him to wait 2 weeks for a consultation followed by another delay for scheduling of further diagnostic testing. I called the pulmonologist, presented the situation, and asked his advice. Did he think this should wait 2 weeks? If not, should the patient be admitted to the hospital for an expedited evaluation, or could he arrange for a same-day evaluation? By offering this range of options, I availed myself of the consultant's expertise while advocating for the patient. The pulmonologist agreed that the constellation of symptoms warranted more urgent evaluation and fit the patient in that day for consultation followed by an expedited bronchoscopy for diagnosis. A consultation with a thoracic surgeon quickly followed, and I breathed a sigh of relief. I felt terrible that the patient had cancer, yet relieved that I had done my best to provide optimal patient care.

There are some patients who would demand the extra service, and there are others who medically deserve it. Knowing the difference and acting upon it makes for outstanding care (see Calibrate your Concern in Chap. 6). Care is the effort we expend to optimize patients' health and well-being. Service encompasses the details that lead to burnout. The key is to strike the balance that protects you and protects your patients. The risk of death dictates the timeline.

10.4 The Person Behind the Patient

Understanding the science of medicine brings great intellectual fulfillment. Knowing the details that make your patient a person brings great emotional fulfillment. Both intellectual and emotional fulfillment are essential to sustain you for a life in medicine. Do your best to embrace, encourage, and celebrate these details. I try to learn a nonmedical fact about every patient I care for; it is these nonmedical facts that strengthen the patient-physician bond.

I have heard the most wonderful stories: the septuagenarian patient and his wife, so visibly in love, that I asked them one day how long they had been married. I must have looked startled when they said, "5 years this month!" as I knew they had children and grandchildren. They told me the story: both were widowed and were regulars at the same coffee shop. The waitress who served them for months set them up on a date, and the rest is (social) history. What a privilege, to have a window into people's lives: encourage the stories that turn patients into people because you will both benefit from the experience.

10.4.1   Embrace the Little Details

There will be times when your schedule doesn't offer the luxury of long stories; there may be more patients waiting to be seen. That's okay, because the social history is the perfect time to efficiently gather special and unique details: where the patient grew up, what they do, how many kids and grandkids. Record personal details in the chart for future reference. For example, "She has 3 grandchildren and fourth on the way, the first boy, due in June." The detailed record-keeping brings you both joy and provides a point of connection at a future visit.

Ask about the names and ages of kids and pets and put the information in the note. This is especially gratifying when I haven't seen a patient in a while, and I ask if Sally is now 5 and Timothy 8; show patients that the details of their lives are important to you. I once saw a patient after a year and asked him how many grandchildren he now had: he said 17. I did a double take because I had recorded, a year prior, that he had 2. Observing my confusion, he laughed and explained that he had remarried 9 months prior and his new wife had 15 grandchildren whom he now counted as his own. We commiserated over the sharp increase in his Christmas gift budget, and I made sure to document and celebrate his new marriage in my note.

There are so many decision points during a patient visit: patients will drop all sorts of clues and it's up to the physician to decide which avenues are the highest diagnostic yield. Not every question has to be aimed at determining the best diagnosis or treatment plan. The non-medical details you learn will strengthen the patient-physician bond. The insight will also help you weigh items in the differential and forge the trust needed to implement your treatment plan. Even more, these details will bring joy to the often routine work of patient care.

10.4.2   Ask the Follow-Up Question

I always ask patients about exercise because it's a high-yield question. A patient who exercises regularly without limitations with no change in energy and endurance over the past year is generally a healthy patient. If a patient reports a departure from their usual exercise program, this may signal a change in their health, perhaps a new cardiovascular or orthopedic limitation that bears further investigation. However, a change in exercise can also offer insight into more than just stamina and endurance—you will uncover important details if you ask the right questions.

A patient once told me he hadn't exercised for the past 6 weeks because he'd been busier than usual. I could have let it go, assuming that it was work occupying his time. Instead, I delved deeper because I had documented, in my note from 6 months prior, that he was jogging 3 miles 5 days/week. It seemed an abrupt shift for someone with a dedicated exercise program. When I asked him what had happened 6 weeks ago to interrupt his usual exercise program, he explained that his wife had been diagnosed with cancer. Since then, he had been consumed with doctors' appointments, chemotherapy sessions, and the caring for her in the aftermath of those sessions.

He had not volunteered the information and seemed relieved to talk about it; I made a note in the chart so I could ask about his wife at future appointments. What if I had just advised him to return to exercise when life calmed down, and not asked what had made him busier 6 weeks prior? I would have missed out on the opportunity to learn more about his life. Part of experience is hearing what the patient doesn't say and encouraging them to elaborate.

Other ways to forge connection: if the patient tells you they stopped smoking on April 6, 2002, there's a story there. Specific dates herald milestones. For one patient, it was the birth of his first child; for another, it was because her boyfriend wouldn't marry her until she quit (when she recounted this story to me, they had been married for decades).

10.4.3   Address the Little Indignities

The Boy Scouts have a rule regarding camp sites: "Always leave it better than you found it." That applies to a patient's room as well. Before you exit, right between "Is there anything I can to do make your life easier?" and leaving, ask about the lights and TV (on or off), tray table location, and door (open or closed). Even in the hospital after a happy and uneventful childbirth, I was sore and exhausted. The thought of having to reorient the tray table overwhelmed me. Multiply that by the mental and physical stress of illness, and the constant interruptions by staff where the patient is forced to politely submit to interrogations and examinations (essential, aimed to help, though nonetheless intrusive), and do your best to make your visit more helpful than stressful.

The next kindness originated with Dr. Bernard Lown, renowned cardiologist and humanitarian, and was passed down through his mentees who later became my mentors. When a patient leans forward so you can listen to their lungs, turn the pillow over to the fresher, cooler side. This has been celebrated by the late, great sportscaster Stuart Scott who had a catchphrase, "Cool as the other side of the pillow". The Germans (of course) even have a word for the refreshing side of a pillow: "*Kissenkühlelabsal*" or "pillow cool refreshment." Whether inspired by Dr. Lown, Stuart Scott, or the idiosyncrasies of the German language, remember this tiny kindness. Small acts of kindness bring happiness to the patient, build trust, and keep your focus where it belongs—on your patients' well-being which is an essential component of their health.

These tiny kindnesses can apply to outpatients as well. Living in Southern California, everyone endures the oppressive weight of heavy traffic. A morning commute can be extended by an extra 15–20 min just by leaving 5 min later if that late start coincides with the morning rush. The distance between locations is measured not in miles, but in minutes.

Due to the traffic, coupled with parking fees at the medical center, try coordinate patient appointments. For example, a patient may need to see the electrophysiologist to discuss defibrillator placement for sudden cardiac death. The appointment is not urgent, and the patient will be back to see you in three months. Work with your office staff to arrange the two appointments on the same day and save the patient an extra trip. A little additional forethought on your part can provide significant benefit to your patients.

10.4.4 Humor

When I was in medical school, an older and highly revered professor gave us a lecture on the patient-physician relationship and told us to never joke around with patients. If you tried to be funny, he warned, the patient would not take you seriously, and it would turn into a contest of who was the funniest. For years afterwards, I was careful to never joke around with my patients.

Then I had a mentor as a cardiology fellow who had the best relationships with his patients—they trusted him implicitly. He would joke with them, when the setting was right, and they loved it. When patients came in for their routine heart biopsies post heart transplantation, feeling great and doing well, the nurse would say, "This doc is awesome! He's been at this for about a week and is such a quick learner!" And my mentor would respond, "Hey, can you hold the instructional manual right side up? I can't read the next step." Now, the patients had experienced countless expert biopsies performed by my mentor, so the humor set the perfect tone and eased any butterflies. They knew they were in the best hands.

The power of humor was not the only revelation here: I realized that the advice of one mentor could contradict that of another and that advice that's relevant at an early career stage may be less helpful later. The patient-physician relationship grows with experience. The medical school mentor's advice was appropriate for me early in my training when I was inexperienced and focusing all my energies on grasping the intricacies of differential diagnosis and management algorithms. With greater experience and stronger relationships with patients, my fellowship mentor's advice rang true. When you have a relationship with a patient, and they trust you, humor is a gift that can bring you closer together. I value the advice I received from both; each had a place in my professional growth.

While I'm no comedian, there are several situations when humor can set the right tone. The first is the healthy cranky patient. I had a patient who grumbled about the frequent blood draws after transplant. I said, "It's wonderful to hear your voice, even when you're complaining, since a few months ago, you were too short of breath to say much!" A little humor refocused the situation and reframed her priorities. She understood the importance of lab draws. At my quip, she smiled, rolled her eyes, and we moved on. Another patient might not have responded so well; it's important to know your patients—read the room.

Humor can also defuse the tension of an otherwise serious discussion—for the right patient, based on their cues. I cared for a heart transplant recipient who had advanced cardiac allograft vasculopathy and warranted consideration of redo transplantation. He was naturally devastated by the news. I told him that we would combat his fear and sadness with a plan. He was grateful to channel his fear and worry into something constructive. He felt weepy and told me that he was glad that I was not. I joked, "Who would want a weepy doctor? Doctors don't weep; doctors make plans!" And at every visit since, leading up to his second transplant and years later, when he was thriving with transplant number 2, he would greet me in clinic, "Is that my weepy doctor?" I would respond, "No weepy docs here— let's go through the plan!" Together, we turned one of the scariest moments in his life into a humorous one—because it was the right approach for him.

Humor is a great antidote to heavy emotions. When a patient is thanking you for saving their life (the best feeling in the world), you don't want to be put on too high a pedestal. In this situation, I usually say, "I know, right? I'm so awesome I can't even believe it! This is the best team in the world and we love taking care of you." Here, humor defuses the strong emotions, turns tears to laughter, and emphasizes that importance of the team. Doctors are not gods, and most of the business of saving lives comes down to effective teamwork. Emphasize your humanity. The patient-physician relationship thrives in the details that make you both human— accepting, sharing, and celebrating them.

10.5   Maintaining Homeostasis

I am lucky to have never been a patient, except during childbirth and I am grateful to describe the experience as all miracle and no disaster. I have never experienced what I have frequently observed in hospitalized patients: the dreary monotony of the days, punctuated by frequent unscheduled interruptions from the medical staff. I sense the pressure patients feel to be polite to everyone who enters the room, even when they are tired, scared, worried, or in pain. The greatest diversion in the day may be the lunch tray (another reason why a late tray is just another straw on the camel's back; see Chap. 12 on Managing Expectations).

Even in the most joyous of occasions, the delivery of a healthy baby, there are situations fraught with stress. I had hypertension after the birth of one of my children. The resident seemed as nervous and unsure of the plan as I was, which only served to further elevate my blood pressure. He was wise enough to return with his senior resident who calmly explained the next steps; she put us both at ease because she had a concrete action plan. The lesson: when you sense your inexperience is impacting your ability to provide the best care, return with experienced reinforcements.

There are other times when a hospitalization goes perfectly. You feel cared for as a person and a patient. My third child was born on the Sunday of the LA marathon. I drove to the hospital just before the street closures began; my obstetrician, Dr. B., wasn't so lucky. He parked in the closest parking space he could find, in a condominium parking lot and, hoping his car wouldn't be towed, jogged four blocks to the hospital to deliver the baby. This incredible dedication gave me even more faith in his competence. Little details make an enormous difference; imagine this magnified exponentially when patients are sick.

I see this most acutely in my patients with advanced heart failure who remain in the hospital awaiting heart transplantation. They are often trapped in bed due to continuous monitoring from a pulmonary artery catheter or support with a temporary mechanical circulatory support device. They are dependent on assistance for even minor tasks like taking a few steps to the bathroom. Their only hope of someday leaving the hospital and living a healthy life is surviving a major risky surgery which could happen in a day, or a month—or never.

Yet every day, when I enter the room on rounds with my team, these patients are invariably smiling. After a quick chat, I move on with my day and they remain trapped in their room waiting for the magic call for the donor heart, a wait both unpredictable (when will it happen?) and uncertain (will it ever happen?). Before exiting, I like to ask, "Is there anything I can do to make your life easier?" Sometimes they joke about ribeye steaks or mani-pedis. Other times, they let me know about the bothersome little things that I can actually fix: vital signs in the middle of the night, monotonous meal trays, constipation, difficulty sleeping.

When someone is in the hospital, especially for the long and unpredictable wait for a heart transplant, bothersome little things become amplified by their frequency and the ever-present weight of uncertainty and fear. While the future may be (possibly, hopefully) bright, it will take a major surgery fraught with risks to get there. While a hospitalization on the heart transplantation waiting list is an extreme example, it's emblematic of the minor indignities all hospitalized patients face.

Based on my experience with these hospitalizations, I aim to maintain quality of life in hospitalized patients by addressing 3 critical factors that govern our homeostasis from birth: eat, poop, and sleep.

10.5.1 Eat

There is nothing magical about NPO after midnight before a surgery or procedure: if the procedure is at 4 pm versus 7 am, does the patient need to fast those additional 9 h? Toddlers and trainees aren't the only ones who get hangry. Instead of making every patient with a planned procedure NPO after midnight, confirm with the physician doing the procedure how many hours of NPO are required and write the order accordingly. For afternoon procedures in the cardiac catheterization laboratory that require conscious sedation, an early light breakfast with no lunch is often fine. The patient will be grateful to have control of at least one homeostatic factor.

There are other considerations regarding food. When patients are tired, during a long hospital stay, of the monotonous cafeteria fare, call a nutrition consult to brainstorm acceptable dietary variations and allow patients to bring in food from home. As I tell my patients awaiting heart transplantation, eat whatever you like—as long as it's low in salt, though even this directive is flexible.

A young woman awaiting heart transplantation was stuck in the hospital on her birthday. She wanted only three things: a Dr. Pepper, dumplings from a Chinese restaurant down the block from the hospital, and her boyfriend to share the meal. With some adjustments in her diuretic dosing and close monitoring of the filling pressures by pulmonary artery catheter, she enjoyed the birthday meal she was craving with no detriment to her hemodynamic parameters. When she was discharged from the hospital after transplantation, her first celebratory meal was the same, with her boyfriend-turned-fiancé included. This time, with the gift of normal cardiac function, no adjustment in diuretics were required.

Finally, fluid restriction. A one-liter fluid restriction is cruel and unusual punishment for a patient with heart failure. If you cannot achieve adequate diuresis with a humane 2-L fluid restriction, then there's something more serious at play than an inadequate diuretic regimen. Instead of fashioning a draconian fluid restriction that's impossible to achieve, investigate other reasons for diuretic resistance: cardiogenic shock or renal dysfunction.

10.5.2 Poop

Constipation is uncomfortable, and constipation begets constipation. While the plural of anecdote is not data, I have observed that constipation can also result in serious morbidity. I had a patient who had constipation so bad it contributed to bowel ischemia for which he ultimately required partial colectomy, and another who strained so hard for a bowel movement early post transplantation while on high-dose steroids that he sustained vertebral compression fractures.

We all know the importance of regular bowel habits. Imagine how difficult must it be to maintain regular bowel movements when you are immobile in the hospital, at the mercy of care assistants to help you to the bedpan or commode, facing the ever-present threat of an interruption from the rounding team. While colace is little more than placebo, regimens from above like Miralax and from below like suppositories can be lifesavers (literally). Ask early, address early, prevent problems. As I tell trainees, "Don't pooh-pooh constipation."

10.5.3 Sleep

I love to sleep. I hate the fact that my patients often cannot sleep in the hospital. There are many sources of insomnia: fear, anxiety, and pain are the hardest to fix and the most important to address. Then there are the littler ones that can be more easily remedied: middle-of-the-night lab draws and vital signs—why? For patients awaiting heart transplantation, I have fashioned a standard order set for no routine vital signs or nursing interruptions between 10 PM and 4 AM, and this can be applied to all patients. (Seems appropriate, as that's about my sleep schedule too.)

Speaking of lab draws: does any patient who is not in diabetic ketoacidosis ever actually need twice daily labs? Challenge yourself by assessing how often you change management based on the evening labs. Think about how you could address the morning labs in such a way that a recheck is not necessary until the next morning. If the potassium is 2.5 mEq/L on the morning draw then a recheck later in the day is essential. What if the potassium is 3.6 mEq/L with normal renal function? Empower yourself to be aggressive in your repletion and check again the next morning.

Consider also how much you dislike having your blood drawn and imagine you are in the hospital where the phlebotomist appears multiple times a day to draw yours. Imagine how you would feel if you knew that the BID lab order was just a knee-jerk without careful assessment of how the second set of daily labs changed management. I hope that after you consider all these issues, you'll pause before ordering twice-daily laboratories again.

What about medications? I have a rule: loop diuretics are never prescribed three times a day (TID). There is essentially no way to fashion a TID regimen to avoid making the patient pee late into the night. Rather, administer high-dose BID diuretic (second dose early afternoon, not 12 h from the first dose). If that doesn't work, prescribe a continuous infusion that's turned off between 10 PM and 4 AM. Are you wondering if these diuretic regimens prolong hospitalization? Isn't every day in the hospital a chance for a patient to fall out of bed and get *C difficile* colitis?

Yes, which means that you should make every *day* count, rather than every night. Be aggressive with your morning dosing so that peeing at night is not necessary. Are you now wondering why I don't just put a Foley catheter in every patient with heart failure? Because indwelling catheters are uncomfortable and increase the risk of infection. Don't rely on a catheter fraught with risk when smart dosing strategies can achieve an optimal outcome without it.

Along this vein (no pun intended), there is no spotting of diuretics in the middle of the night. If the patient has not met their I/O goal but is hemodynamically stable and not in respiratory distress, they should not have to pay for your inability to diurese them during the day by peeing all night. This is yet another reason to be aggressive during the day and eliminate the night float's nighttime I/O rounds.

10.6 Final Thoughts

The strategies outlined in this chapter follow certain themes: see your patient as a person and empathize—imagine what it feels like to be a patient. The former strategy will strengthen the patient-physician bond and bring joy to the practice of medicine. The latter strategy will help you to do your best to ease the stress, fear, and uncertainty of medical care.

Chapter 11
Being a Woman in Medicine (Men: Don't Skip This Chapter!)

I was raised on 3 immutable truths: first, I would become the fifth generation of physicians in my family; second, as a woman, I would be a minority in medicine; and third, I would have to work twice as hard as a man to be considered one-half as good. In grade school, I wondered if my parents' dour view of women in the workplace was overly pessimistic. By the time I completed fellowship, I realized it was partially true. Nearly 50% of all US medical school students are female, but as of 2016, only 12% of board-certified cardiologists are women (Mehta et al 2019). I am one of the 12%. In the two decades since I graduated from medical school, I have been treated differently because I'm a woman. From these experiences, I've learned to navigate the challenges of the training environment, motherhood, and career.

An important note before we begin: the strategies and challenges described below apply to the hurtful microaggressions prevalent in medical training and beyond. I am fortunate to have never experienced the darker side of sexual harassment in my career. For those who have survived this, my advice is always: tell your mentor early and often and if your mentor is not responsive, escalate your concern up the chain of command in your program or department including discussions with Human Resources. Sexual harassment or aggression is abhorrent and must be met with zero tolerance and swift action.

11.1 Navigating the Training Environment

11.1.1 Never Assume the Worst

As a third-year medical student on my surgical rotation, I knew the drill. On vascular surgery rounds, keep the bag packed with gauze and tape for dressing changes on rounds. On neurosurgery, prep the intern's notes. In the operating room, place the Foley catheter in the anesthetized patient.

I was ready, then, when the senior surgical resident said, "Hey, Michelle, the patient's asleep. Time to place the Foley!" I had never placed a Foley catheter in a woman before. When I timidly admitted this, he said, "You know the anatomy. Figure it out!" I scurried off, chastened, and begged the scrub nurse to help me. Fortunately, she did.

Years later, I wondered if I misread the incident. Was he being condescending because of my sex, or sarcastic because I was lower on the training totem pole? Did he mean that I should know the anatomy because I was a woman, or because I was a diligent medical student? Would he have spoken to male medical student that way? I'm not a mind reader; I'll never know for sure. I chose to believe that his rude behavior was inspired by my station and not my sex; how many women without medical training can locate the urethra anyway?

I didn't report him at the time because it didn't occur to me to be insulted. I felt embarrassed that I didn't know the anatomy and worked harder. Besides this remark, he was a great resident. He taught me how to identify a pleural effusion on a decubitus film, why any organ that exhibits peristalsis can cause colicky pain, how chest tubes work. If I had reported him, maybe he would have reined in the rare sarcastic comments. On the other hand, maybe he would have been less eager to volunteer his time to teach medical students for fear of reprisal for offhand remarks.

There was no decision to make at the time because the gender-insensitive nature of his comment did not register. Now, through the lens of retrospect, I see how his words could have been misconstrued. I would never make a remark this like to a resident, male or female. Still, I did not jump to the conclusion of assuming the worst. He was otherwise supportive and even encouraged me to pursue a career in surgery. This rude incident was an outlier in an otherwise unblemished trend of supportive behavior.

This principle, to try to assume to the best, also applies to patients. I have been called "sweetie" and "honey" more times than I can count. One patient always called me his "16-year-old doctor." I cared for him for over a decade, through a valve replacement, progressive heart failure, heart transplantation, and ultimately hospice care. While he would always greet me with a joke about my age, he also sought my advice with every medical decision, requested me for all his angiograms, and only agreed to hospice after I told him that I understood and supported his decision. His comments about my youthful appearance taken in the context of a decade of trust were charming, not belittling. He taught me to consider the context more than the label, and to begin by assuming the best—or at least, not the worst.

I have so many stories like this: whenever I enter the exam room, there is a patient who always stands, hugs me, and says, "Miss Michelle, it's wonderful to see you!" He proceeds to sit down and give me his rapt attention. He follows my explanations with interest, never questions my judgment, and often ends the visit by thanking me for saving his life.

What would be the point of correcting the "Miss Michelle?" It would embarrass him and hurt his feelings without any upside for me. I suppose you could argue that if I were to say something, he will not make the same mistake with other women physicians. I would counter that it's not a mistake; it's just a courtly gentleman showing affection for his physician. Context matters and meeting his kindness with antagonism would harm our relationship. Sometimes, I resort to humor and say, smiling, "You know I'm married, right? So 'Mrs. Michelle' or 'Dr. Michelle' will do." Other times, I just accept his hug.

On the other hand, there are other patients for whom addressing you by your first name is just the tip of the iceberg of disrespect. They will call you by your first name to let you know that they do not value your judgment or expertise. While I rarely focus solely on the mode of address, I will call such patients out on their behavior. I will address the elephant in the room: "You seem uncomfortable with my care. Let's talk about why. If you'd rather not, let's find you a physician who might be a better fit." Of course, "better fit" generally refers to a demographic distinct from my own.

While I call out the disrespect, I rarely address the (first) name-calling. My sense is the patient is doing it to get under my skin, so what better response than no response at all? Even if I did address it, they would likely not see the error of their ways and instead become defensive. There may be satisfaction in direct confrontation, though it would not achieve the ultimate goal of providing optimal care. I focus on what I can do to improve their health (find them a doctor they can trust), because I'm unlikely to fix their personality.

The biggest lessons here: (1) context is more important than labels; and (2) when the context is the problem, focus on how you can still promote optimal patient care.

11.1.2 Claim Your Role

As an intern in the medical ICU, the nurses rarely took me seriously. When a patient had a temperature of 103 and rigors, I would say, "Let's start a fluid bolus? And draw blood cultures?" Inevitably, the nurse's eyes would shift up and to the side, to my resident standing next to me, for confirmation. I inwardly fumed every time this happened. I knew how to work up sepsis; I didn't need to be second-guessed just because I was a diminutive Indian woman. Yet there were other female interns who looked like me who weren't treated like me.

One female surgical intern, also slight, also Asian, was never questioned by the nurses. Intrigued, I surreptitiously monitored her behavior. She was unfailingly polite though never exhibited the slightest upward inflection. I was using the upward inflection of inexperience. While I might have felt confident, I did not sound confident. I needed to make the transition from inexperience to experience in my actions as I had in my thoughts. This surgical intern became an unwitting and fleeting mentor. On my next MICU rotation, I adopted her monotone, and the transformation was dramatic. The nurses listened to me without silently confirming the plan with my resident over my shoulder. I'm not the first person to discover that upward inflections make people take you less seriously. The revelation here: it wasn't my gender, which I couldn't control, but my inflection, which I could, that set the tone for my encounters.

This has served me well as an attending physician. When I walk in the room with the rounding entourage, I'm often the shortest person in the room. I'll introduce myself to the patient as "Dr. Kittleson, the boss of this team!" Patients have a hard enough time deciphering the roles of all the people entering their room; make it easier by claiming your role.

11.1.3 Humor and Sarcasm Can Help

There are times when humor and sarcasm are the best way to deflect the inevitable comments. Patients can be suspicious of a youthful female cardiologist. I don't blame them for being surprised that I am the cardiologist and not the nurse. Since 91% of nurses are female and only 12% of cardiologists are female, probability is on their side if they guess I'm a nurse. I try to see it from a patient's perspective: wouldn't I be surprised if I walked into a nail salon and the manicurist was an old white man? (In fact, 17% of nail technicians are men and 34% are White, so it stands to reason that patients should be as surprised to encounter a female cardiologist as I would be to receive a pedicure from a white man). I forgive the profiling, though it rankles.

For the harmless comments, humor and sarcasm work well. "But you look too young to be a doctor!" is met with "Thank you, my plastic surgeon will be so pleased!" or "You know, insurance plans in Los Angeles cover Botox!" Comments like "But I thought you were the nurse?" merit responses like "It's the strangest thing! In the twenty-first century, women can be doctors too!".

For disrespectful comments, or those laden with distrust and suspicion, humor and sarcasm will not be enough. I'll employ the direct approach outlined above. This is a win–win situation: the patients who trust me, stay with me, and the patients who don't find someone they do. (And a bonus: when the older/White/male cardiologist supports my recommendations, the patient often realizes that competent physicians come in both sexes and I may have smoothed the way for their next female physician.)

11.2 Motherhood (Parenthood)

I have attended many panels on being a woman professional. In college, there was a female astronomer who told the impressionable and wide-eyed contingent of undergraduates that she decided to not get married or have a family because her career would suffer. Her bold proclamation was met with equal parts horror and disbelief. There were plenty of subtle eye rolls since, as freshman on the precipice of our college careers, we were all invincible and ready to have it all.

On another panel, this time in medical school, a surgeon with twins described how she loved the competence and control she felt in the hospital while at home, she was disorganized and harried. One anecdote left me cringing even as I laughed: when her twins were about a year old, this surgeon noticed that she could never seem to find the right outfit for work; something was always missing. After a few more months, she picked up on the pattern: only about half the suits her nanny dropped off at the dry cleaners ended up back in her closet. By the time she figured it out, a significant portion of her wardrobe was unaccounted for, and her nanny had since quit.

She never discovered what her nanny did with those missing suits: did she sell them on eBay, or wear them herself? This surgeon could make split-second life-and-death decisions in the pressure cooker of an operating room yet not keep track of her professional attire. My reaction was again a mix of horror and disbelief; that would never happen to me. I was certain that I would handle motherhood as capably as I had handled medical training.

Those were famous last words. Being a physician is hard. Being a parent is hard. Still, you can be both a physician and a parent, simultaneously, without permanent damage to your career or your wardrobe.

11.2.1 What You Need to Successfully Parent as a Physician

A mentor once shared her three criteria for success being a physician and a parent, noting that two of the three were essential: (1) a supportive partner; (2) family help; and/or (3) dependable and flexible paid childcare. It takes a village to raise a child, and more so in our current world of hyper-scheduling: successfully managing school, playdates, sports and music lessons, pediatrician and dentist appointments requires spreadsheets and family calendars and offerings to the traffic gods.

The supportive partner is key. In every relationship, unless there is unlimited assistance from family and/or paid childcare, someone's career will take a backseat. Someone will have to be more flexible, missing meetings or conferences or late shifts, and this sacrifice may manifest in slower professional advancement or reduced compensation. That's okay if both parties agree to, understand, and appreciate the sacrifice. And there can and should be back-and-forth, where one career can be placed on the back burner for a time and then the other.

Help is crucial. Two working parents, or even one working parent with a stay-at-home partner, can manage the 24–7 demands of childcare, though it will not be easy. Unlike nights in the ICU, parenthood does not come with sick call or moonlighting bonus or duty-hour limits. Having support to relieve you and your partner is critical. Sometimes family can pitch in. Sometimes paid childcare does the trick. Whatever it might be, expect that you will need help and plan for this.

11.2.2 The Right Time to Have Kids

When is the right time to have kids? Now—or never. There will never be a right time—or a wrong time—and nature probably won't cooperate with your schedule anyway. If you're younger, you may have less flexibility and financial freedom, though your knees will creak less after playing hide and seek. If you're older, you may have accrued the seniority to fashion a more flexible career. Still, the stakes of a career slowdown may be higher later on in life and you may have issues with infertility. Having a child is a little like performing a lumbar puncture: if you're wondering if you need one, it's probably time to get one.

The greatest fears I hear from new moms (and dads, though mostly moms) is that they will not be the same physician after they return from parental leave. They worry that they won't be as good or won't love medicine as much as they used to. I had the same fears. While there may be rare exceptions, those parents who fall so in love with parenthood that they don't want to return to being a physician, this fear is mostly unfounded.

11.2.3   Unfounded Fear 1: You Won't Remember How to Be a Good Physician

With each of my three kids, I both dreaded returning to work and couldn't wait to go back. Between the sleep deprivation and constant nursing and needy toddlers, I craved the relative serenity of the hospital. At work, I knew what was expected of me and how to meet those expectations. My fellows were fully potty-trained, didn't throw tantrums, and I never had to repeat a question 7 times before they would answer me. On the other hand, I was worried: would I remember how to deftly manage cardiogenic shock, knowing when to transition from inotropic support to an intra-aortic balloon pump in a decompensating patient? Would I remember how to troubleshoot tricky endomyocardial biopsies from the left internal jugular vein? What would I do when patients showed up late and I didn't have time to pump?

I took great comfort from my mom's experience. She was a pathology resident when I was born and had a harrowing delivery with eclampsia. She was convinced that the pre-delivery seizures had left her with brain damage and was too scared to tell her program director. On her first day back, he asked her to read a set of slides. After she correctly interpreted all of them, he told her it had been a test—not for him, but for her. He picked tricky cases to show her that her rocky delivery and new motherhood had not impacted her clinical skills. Even though she had not voiced her concerns about her competence, he sensed her newfound lack of confidence and devised the best strategy to rebuild it. I love the story for the sensitive and perceptive mentor and the lesson: parenthood is not a distraction that will make you a worse doctor.

The lessons you learn from caring for children can make you a better doctor. You will learn to face anger, obstinance, and frustration with patience and kindness. You will gain compassion as you identify with family members suffering through their loved ones' illnesses. Can you be an amazing doctor without kids? Of course. Can you use the lessons of parenthood to your professional advantage? Absolutely.

11.2.4 Unfounded Fear 2: Your Baby Will Forget You

Let's be frank: with all due respect to pediatricians out there, newborns are blobs who eat, poop, cry, sleep. You will spend your days worrying that these homeostatic functions are either excessive or inadequate. As the days and nights blend into a haze of spit-up and sleep deprivation, you will feel like being a parent is all work and no fun. For the first few months, you're right. Parenthood becomes more fun once the baby can focus on you, then smile, then laugh. However, in the early weeks and months, babies don't really need you. Babies need an attentive warm body—and you will ensure this will be provided for them.

It continues to amaze me: even though I spent the least amount of time with my kids when they were babies: an hour in the morning, a few hours in the evening, moments in the middle of the night, we still shared an incredible connection that only strengthened as they grew. The mantra of '80 s parents, quality time is more important than quantity of time, is true and the daily grind of the parental routines breeds closeness. (My husband and I, latch-key Gen-Xers, never wanted to be helicopter parents.) Your babies will not forget you. Your babies will grow into kids who love you. Leaving your newborn is much harder for you than it is for them. Let's face it: there's not much interaction to be had with a newborn. Warm body plus warm milk plus tight swaddle equals a happy newborn.

11.2.5 Unfounded Fear 3: You Will Never "Get It Together"

In some ways, there will never be balance. Being a parent means you learn to live with your heart permanently outside your body, and you're only as happy as your unhappiest child. Nonetheless, you will achieve predictability and establish a routine where you will remember what it feels like to love your job and also love being a parent.

With each of my 3 kids, I felt my brain waking up when they turned one. By then, I was comfortable with parenting, sleep cycles were better established, and I was no longer pumping every 3–4 h at work. Of course, that's often when the next pregnancy begins, so there will be a cycle of pregnancy-then-baby that may repeat multiple times before you can truly come up for air. Don't despair, though: you will soon enter the Golden Age of Parenting, which I define by 3 criteria: no naps, no diapers, and no teenagers. Look forward to the Golden Age when life will improve.

Let's recap: many of your fears about being a parent and a physician are unfounded: (1) time away from medicine will not make you forget everything you know; (2) when you return to work, your baby will not forget you and will still love you; and (3) after the overwhelming early period of caring for a baby, you will regain a balance where you will derive joy and fulfillment from both your job and your family.

11.3   Navigating the Career

A talented young cardiology fellow approached me one day. She was a research superstar: she had published two major manuscripts in important journals and then, a few months later, delivered a beautiful healthy baby. She had been working on a grant application before the baby was born and it had stalled. When she approached me, she was so worried and hesitant that I thought she was about to break bad news about her health, or her baby's health.

In fact, the bombshell was not the bad news I expected. She was considering taking a break from research and focusing solely on patient care for a few years. While she had loved research, the lack of structure and defined endpoints felt too stressful, and that stress made it difficult for her to enjoy her time away from work with her baby. She wanted to enjoy the regular routine of clinical medicine without the uncertainty of grant applications and manuscripts. She was worried about reception her decision would receive.

I saw myself in this young cardiologist. I had felt the same way when I had my first baby, and I was similarly nervous about telling my mentor that I wanted to take a step back from research. What a difference a few years of experience makes; I was delighted to have the opportunity to show her the same support and encouragement my mentor had shown me.

The relief on her face told me she had not expected this support: I told her that I admired her careful self-reflection and respected and supported her decision. You can "do it all," but not necessarily all at the same time. Life happens in stages, and it's reasonable (better in fact), to figure out what you can and should concentrate on and when. The key is to find colleagues who can mentor you on work-life balance, those who have taken similar paths and can offer support, advice, and encouragement along the way. Here are some of my tips.

11.3.1   *Your Priorities Are Right Because They're Yours*

I had a steady increase in research productivity, as measured by PubMed citations, from the end of residency to 6 years into my first faculty position. For the next 6 years, I had no first-author publications. Why? I spent those years is the fog of pregnancy and caring for a newborn, times 3. Though I kept my patients alive, and I kept my kids alive, I had no desire to do anything else. I am proud that as I turned away research opportunities, I reliably provided optimal patient care. I'm lucky because I had the foresight to choose a job where research productivity was not required. I was fortunate to have a supportive boss who put no pressure on me to publish. Because of this support, I felt comfortable saying no to extras like research projects which, at the time, filled me with dread, not joy.

In 2018, when my youngest turned 1, I felt my mind unfurling. Research ideas now held interest and promise. I gradually re-entered the academic workforce, on my own terms, not because I had to, but because I wanted to. Did taking these years off delay my professional advancement? Maybe. Does this possibility trouble me? Not at all. How much worse it would have been to slog through research I didn't enjoy, just for the sake of doing it. I'm glad I never had to feel as if I were expending the precious and scarce resource of my energy and stamina on manuscript revisions rather than on my family, or on sleep.

Know what your priorities are and recognize that as a physician, caring for your patients and caring for your family should always be at the top of the list. If managing these non-negotiables seems overwhelming, re-assign your other responsibilities. Don't second-guess a decision to focus on family over the rigors of career extras if your heart isn't in the career extras. You may return to research later or find other passions. Embrace what's important and don't apologize for your priorities.

11.3.2 Comparison is the Thief of Joy

I had a colleague in fellowship who did the medical equivalent of envy-scrolling on social media: he would routinely search his colleagues and collaborators on PubMed to see if they had more publications than he did. He would assess their publications by year, journal priority, author order, and type of article. He stopped short of inputting the data into a spreadsheet (I think). He used this mental count as impetus to work harder. That compulsive competitive spirit may have worked for him, though I'm not sure his productivity was worth the misery. Like everything in life, it's best to keep your ego in check.

My advice: don't compare yourself to those amazing former co-fellows of yours who publish 10 manuscripts a year as senior author while you are maybe a middle author on one or two. If research was a passion, and it becomes one again, there are ways to re-enter the research arena. Your goals are not your colleagues' goals. Trying meet your colleagues' goals instead of your own will only end in frustration. Follow your own path to achieve the ultimate goal of optimal patient care.

11.3.3 There is More to Academic Medicine Than Research

When I graduated from fellowship, I was convinced that I would spend the next three decades doing exactly the same thing until I retired. Now, I know that's not true. First of all, I'll definitely be working more than three decades because raising three kids in Southern California is expensive. Second, there are so many ways to reinvent one's career and discover new-found passions in medicine. I always loved medical education, though never expected I would create a popular platform on Twitter to share medical pearls. I always loved poems and medical essays though never imaged that I would write my own.

As your career progresses and experience replaces uncertainty, you will have more energy to discover new passions and rediscover old ones. When family responsibilities are more manageable, you may yearn to make an impact in ways other than direct patient care. There are many directions in which you can take your career. You may have a passion for administrative leadership, education, community service, or renew your interest in non-medical fields. Medicine (and life) continues to be a journey of self-discovery. Re-invention is possible long after your training is complete.

11.4   Final Thoughts

From the training environment to motherhood to career, there will always be challenges for women in medicine. Have the strength of your convictions; believe in your competence. Seek out role models to be your mentors. Face the challenges as opportunities to make you a better physician and a better person.

Reference

Mehta LS, Fisher K, Rzeszut AK, Lipner R, Mitchell S, Dill M, Acosta D, Oetgen WJ, Douglas PS. Current demographic status of cardiologists in the United States. JAMA Cardiol. 2019,4.1029–33.

Chapter 12
Self-Care

12.1 Boundaries

I attended Cardiology Grand Rounds as a fellow and the topic was the amazing Helen Taussig. Dr. Taussig was a pioneer in the field of congenital heart disease, advancing surgical therapies including the Blalock-Taussig shunt for hypoplastic left heart disease. The speaker showed a letter from Dr. Taussig to Dr. Adrian Kantrowitz, a renowned cardiothoracic surgeon, dated February 26, 1968 (Helen 1968). Dr. Taussig wrote, "Thank you for your long and detailed letter which greeted me on my return from winter vacation."

Dr. Taussig's response offered no apology for the delay in her response or desire to hide the reason, a vacation. While Dr. Taussig might have retired from official duties at Johns Hopkins in 1963, her career was far from over when she wrote this letter in 1968. In 1964 President Lyndon Johnson presented her with the Medal of Freedom for her work in the treatment and prevention of children's heart disease. In 1965, she became the first woman to serve as president of the American Heart Association. When she wrote this letter, in 1968, she was not playing shuffleboard in a retirement community. She still ran an active research program. Despite her importance and influence and dedication, she did not apologize for being on vacation; she maintained boundaries.

12.1.1 Vacation Time

Contrast that with a trend over the past decade where email out-of-office auto-replies, instead of stating, "I'm on vacation and will respond to your email when I return" now say "I'm away from the medical center with limited email access." Though the shift may be subtle, to me it connotes a certain embarrassment people have with admitting that they (gasp) have the temerity (or weakness) to take a vacation.

© The Author(s), under exclusive license to Springer Nature Switzerland AG 2022   167
M. Kittleson, *Mastering the Art of Patient Care*,
https://doi.org/10.1007/978-3-031-20920-8_12

In response to this trend, my email auto-reply will go something like this: "Thank you for your email! I'm enjoying a wonderful family vacation and don't despair; I'll check email daily. If that turnaround isn't fast enough for you, please call my office!" When the vacation falls around the holidays, I'll often include a favorite recipe. I adopt this aggressively cheerful tone because I delight in emphasizing the importance of vacation time. I receive so much positive feedback on my vacation auto-replies. I hope they may encourage others to similarly celebrate vacations without apology.

Now, you might quibble with the fact that my auto-reply indicates that I check email daily on vacation. For me, that's a healthy balance. I would rather triage issues for a few minutes daily than return to a deluge of emails when the vacation is over. The anticipatory dread of the email avalanche would ruin my vacation. That's just my personality as an anti-procrastinator: a little work every day is better than a mountain of work at the end.

On the other end of the spectrum, I have a colleague who creates an email rule so every email that arrives during the days he's on vacation is immediately deleted. His auto-reply warns senders of this vanguard practice: "Thanks for your email. To preserve my sanity, it will be deleted so please email me again on ____ so I can address your concerns when I return from vacation." Clearly, he has nerves of steel; you will figure out what system works best for you.

12.1.2   100% Care Does Not Require 100% Access

Embracing the importance of vacation time is only one way to create boundaries. It is also necessary to create boundaries with patients. There are patients who want 100% access to me, my cell phone number, my presence in the operating room during their surgery, same-day appointments for any concern. When a patient makes a request like this, the first question I ask myself is: Does optimal patient care require this level of attention? If the answer is no, then I will explain why.

I do not give out my cell phone for many reasons: I have outstanding partners, keep meticulous records, and cannot provide the optimal patient care without a healthy balance of rest and family time. I will not be in the operating room because the anesthesiologist is highly trained to perform cardiac monitoring and my presence would be superfluous at best and distracting at worst. My unnecessary presence in the operating room would also prevent me from caring for patients who truly require my expertise. I do not universally offer same-day appointments because not every concern warrants this urgency. There is a difference between medical urgency and a patient's desire for urgency. If I were to indulge urgent requests that are not medically warranted, then patients who have medical indications for urgent evaluation would have delays in their care.

Patients accept these explanations. What they really want, I have found, when they ask for my cell phone or presence in the operating room or the promise of same-day appointments, is just to know that they can rely on me to provide the best care to them. The question is "How I can reach you 24–7?" The "emotion behind the question" is fear. Patients are really asking, "Are you paying attention to me? Do you care about me? Will you be there for me?" When I address the emotion behind the question, explaining that I will always triage their concerns appropriately, patients visibly relax.

12.2 Patient Reviews

An enormous part of self-care is not reading patient reviews. I escaped these for years, until my medical center adopted the anonymous patient experience telephone surveys, and the results were deposited in my inbox every month. When I received my first report from the survey, I skimmed over the glowing comments about how I was the best doctor ever. All I could focus on was the one patient who gave me an overall rating of 3 out of 10. The patient wrote: "The doctor didn't go over any of the paperwork that I was asked to complete... including my medical history that was all ignored, that bothered me."

Equipped with the encounter date provided and my powers of deduction, I figured out his identity and reviewed the chart because I wanted to know where I went wrong. I was the fifth cardiologist he had seen in two years. Before his visit, I pored over records from all 4 prior cardiologists. His doctor-shopping made him complicated though his medical issues were straightforward.

I counseled him that his anxiety about his condition was impacting his quality of life more than the condition itself and advised him to discuss strategies to manage anxiety with his internist. I did not tell him what he wanted to hear: that I had discovered a problem with his heart that I could fix and resolve his symptoms. Rather, I told him what he needed to hear: his heart was not the problem. He expressed his appreciation in person and then delivered a scathing review via the anonymous telephone survey a few days later.

I was blindsided and there was nothing I could do. Rather than constructive criticism, his review felt like a comment on Yelp, where anonymous users can post reviews, both constructive and cruel, with impunity.

After reading his review, I had fleeting and unwelcome thoughts with subsequent patient encounters: what might the patient say in the survey? I had internal conversations during clinic visits, defending my care even as I delivered it. The worst part was the feeling that my patients and I were not always allies in their health; through the machinations of an anonymous survey, we could become adversaries.

When I read that review, I had already been in practice over a decade with many successes and accolades to my credit. Yet just one bad review resulted in niggling self-doubt and an unwelcome dent in my confidence, hard-won through years of training and practice. If as an experienced physician, I could be so affected by anonymous negative reviews, imagine the devastating impact on newly minted physicians.

A newly minted pediatrician told me that she was nervous to recommend the HPV vaccine to her patients because a parent complained that by doing so, she was promoting promiscuity. A family medicine physician told me that he no longer listed obesity on the patient's problem list as a patient told him this was rude and insulting. This was a patient with multiple obesity-related complications who he felt would benefit from bariatric surgery, yet he was unsure whether his medical recommendations would be met with gratitude or condemnation. An obstetrician told me that she performed a Cesarean section whenever requested, even if a trial of labor would be medically preferable, as she feared the negative consequences of not acquiescing to the mother's birth plan.

Attending physicians fresh out of training fear missing diagnoses, choosing the wrong management strategy, and failing to form therapeutic relationships with their patients. They require time to craft styles of practice. Though capable, they may be tentative and uncertain. Negative comments without context cannot make them better physicians. Negative comments without context will serve only to strip away their confidence when they need it most.

Let me be clear: patients should be satisfied with their care. Patients should trust that their physicians' only priority is optimal patient care and patients should be confident that their physicians have the skills to provide this. Trust and confidence are the cornerstones of the patient-physician relationship. This relationship is not science; it is an art. It cannot be defined, evaluated, or improved upon by an anonymous multiple-choice survey.

Let me also be clear: patients must have recourse when they are dissatisfied with their physician's care. However, that recourse has more than one purpose. Anonymous feedback may be satisfying to the patient in the short-term—patients can vent and have their say. However, in the long-term, this cursory feedback will not improve their care or that of future patients.

Could there be a system to achieve both these goals: the patient is heard, and care is improved? I know the answer is yes because I chair the Peer Review Committee at my medical center. If an issue with the quality of patient care is identified, whether by a patient or by a health care professional, the Peer Review Committee receives a notification. Members of the committee, physicians at the medical center, review the patient's concerns. The committee then decides whether a lapse in care occurred and what strategies could prevent such a lapse in the future. The physician involved receives written guidance and specific suggestions for improvement while the patient source remains anonymous.

A few years ago, I reviewed the case of a patient who presented to urgent care with chest pain, nausea, and vomiting. The urgent care physician ordered sublingual nitroglycerin. Fortunately, before administering it, the nurse realized reviewed the patient's medications and discovered that he had taken sildenafil for erectile dysfunction a few hours prior. This careful and conscientious action might have saved the patient's life; hypotension from nitroglycerin plus sildenafil in a patient with unstable angina could have had fatal consequences. The medical director of urgent care brought the case to the attention of the Peer Review Committee. The case provided an opportunity to provide specific feedback to the physician as well as a general education to the department about the importance of medication reconciliation prior to administration of nitroglycerin.

On another occasion, an office manager asked the Peer Review Committee to review the practice of a physician with multiple patient complaints. Patients reported that they never received feedback on bloodwork checked at their visits. On a number of occasions, issues remained unaddressed, including anemia requiring further diagnostic assessment, hyperlipidemia warranting statin therapy, and hyperkalemia meriting adjustment in antihypertensive medications. When the Peer Review Committee brought these issues to the physician's attention, he was relieved: he was suffering from significant personal stress and needed support to maintain his practice. The Peer Review Committee was able to connect him with support for his personal stress and practice; he was grateful and his patient care improved.

Anonymous telephone surveys involve less time, energy, and resources than Peer Review Committees. The former allows health care administrators to pore over metrics, tie those metrics to compensation, and construct enticing marketing websites. The latter can help physicians and patients improve their practice and provide optimal patient care together.

After that first fateful survey summary landed in my inbox, I have not read another. It is human nature to forget the many laudatory comments and focus on the negative few. The anonymous nature of these reviews does not allow me to improve my practice; it just makes me second-guess myself as I do my best to care for patients. If a good review comes from telling patients what they want to hear rather than what they need to hear, I'll suffer a bad review. The patient's health must be paramount. Otherwise, what are we all doing here? Explain your recommendations with compassion and confidence in your expertise. Prioritize the patient's health before satisfaction scores; this is the best way to optimize patient care, and self-care.

12.3 Grief and Mistakes

As a cardiologist specializing in advanced heart failure and transplantation, I have saved lives and witnessed plenty of tragedy. For years, I lay awake at night grieving the losses and this grief had nowhere to go. To process the grief and move on, I have fashioned stages:

(1) Separate fault from fluke,
(2) Distinguish the unforeseen from the expected,
(3) Accept that control is an illusion.

12.3.1 Separate Fault from Fluke

As a cardiology fellow, I cared for a patient with a mechanical aortic and mitral valves who underwent pacemaker placement. The next morning, she was bradycardic and hypotensive. I spent precious minutes checking an echocardiogram to assess for pericardial effusion (the wrong move, as tamponade would cause tachycardia, of course) when she had a myocardial infarction caused by an embolus down the right coronary artery.

She passed away after heroic resuscitation efforts and I replayed her case at 2 o'clock in the morning for weeks afterward. If I had not wasted time with the echocardiogram, would she have survived? Probably not—though I'll never know. Eventually, I learned to sleep through the night again, mainly because sleep cannot elude the exhausted cardiology fellow forever, and also because I resolved that her death would make me a better doctor. I'll never forget that a coronary embolus can occur in patients with mechanical valves, and a few years later, I made this unusual diagnosis, and the patient lived.

The first step, continued: if, after conversations with trusted mentors, you can establish that the bad outcome was not your fault, resolve not to change your practice based on it; so-called "doctoring by anecdote." I knew a cardiologist who never prescribed sedation before an angiogram because one patient (with radiation-included severe aortic stenosis and left main coronary artery disease) had a cardiac arrest after administration of midazolam and fentanyl.

When I referred patients to him for coronary intervention, they would complain bitterly about their uncomfortable experiences in the cardiac catheterization laboratory. I asked him why he made the experience so uncomfortable; I challenged him to justify why patients without severe aortic stenosis or critical coronary artery disease should be denied sedative medications. He explained that he never wanted another patient to have a cardiac arrest in the cardiac catheterization laboratory. This was a lofty yet unrealistic goal. As the aphorism goes, "If you don't experience complications, it means you're not doing enough cases." He allowed grief and fear to make him a worse doctor instead of a better one. He was trapped in inexperience. Doctor by guidelines, doctor by clinical trials, and doctor by experience—don't allow bad outcomes to motivate you to doctor by anecdote.

12.3.2   Distinguish the Unforeseen from the Expected

While bad outcomes are always horrible, unexpected bad outcomes are worse. (This is one of many reasons why I hold obstetricians in the highest regard; giving birth appears to me equal parts miracle and imminent disaster.) In the high-stakes world of advanced heart failure, patients by dint of walking into my office have a dismal 1-year life expectancy. However, that doesn't mean that they, or their families, understand that tragedy can strike at any moment.

A patient with advanced heart failure saw me because his local center considered him too complex for transplantation. He flew across the country, anticipating that in a few months, he would be home with a new heart. Instead, he decompensated. Faced with few options, he underwent placement of a total artificial heart. Despite the decompensation, I maintained an optimistic focus. I explained that once he had recovered from the surgery to implant the total artificial heart, he would be listed for heart transplantation at a high urgency status. Then, after a projected short wait time, the plan would remain the same: get a heart transplant, recover, recuperate for a few months near our center and then fly back home to his family.

My optimism was tragically misplaced. After the surgery to place the total artificial heart, he never left the intensive care unit. He spent months battling sepsis, renal failure, gastrointestinal bleeding, and respiratory failure. Finally, he suffered a massive stroke and he died in our intensive care unit, far from home, with only his wife at his bedside.

At the end, I found it difficult to look his wife in the eye, though I forced myself to visit his bedside daily. I never had the courage to ask his wife: if I had better prepared them for this potential tragic outcome, if I had described the possibility of a painful death far from home, would he have acquiesced to placement of the total artificial heart? I think he would have; after all, in the midst of a decompensation, he had no other options for survival to transplantation. Still, the fact that my explanation would not have changed the outcome was besides the point. This was not a failure of medical decision-making; this was a failure of preparation.

I failed him, not because he died, but because he was not prepared for it. I felt the grief of his death more acutely because I knew that I could have done better. Now, I do my best to courageously confront bad news. Medical training should include strategies to prepare patients for bad outcomes. Do your best to prepare patients and their families for the worst-case scenarios.

12.3.3 Accept that Control is an Illusion

Sometimes, when something awful happens, the right answer is not to shoulder the responsibility—it is simply to carry on. I cared for a young woman placed on extracorporeal membrane oxygenation after sudden cardiac death. She developed multisystem organ failure and an ischemic leg requiring amputation. At daily family meetings, her father took meticulous notes, as if knowledge could reverse her downward spiral. It did not, and she died.

When I exited the family meeting at which we discussed the withdrawal of life-prolonging interventions, my mind was sluggish with grief. Shortly thereafter, a healthy outpatient cornered me in the corridor. She complained that my office hadn't faxed records to her internist; a stark reminder that I did not have the privilege of grief. I was not the proximate cause to this young woman's death and I had done everything I could to prepare her family; I gave myself permission to let it go. Holding on to your grief helps no one, least of all other patients who need your help.

12.3.4   Learn from Your Successes Too

A codicil: when you make an amazing diagnosis, bask in the warm glow of success, and then figure out how it happened. I consulted on a patient status post knee replacement with a near-syncopal episode. There was a right-sided S3 gallop and a V/Q scan showed multiple pulmonary emboli. When you make a save, be proud. When you learn from the save, recognize that you are crossing the bridge from inexperience to experience.

I listened for right-sided S3 gallops on every patient after that, though the real lesson was to listen to my gut. A minimizer by nature, I would have written off the patient's near-syncope as hypovolemia or a vasovagal reaction to post-operative pain. I didn't write it off because his fear and agitation made me uncomfortable. That was the lesson, to pay attention to that prickly sensation of things not falling neatly into place, and to dig deeper to find the source.

My heart has been broken countless times by tragic outcomes. Maintain your stamina for the many patient-years ahead by processing tragedy as a doctor and not as a loved one. Separating fault from fluke, distinguishing the unforeseen from the expected, and accepting that control is an illusion will help you to become a better doctor and a better person. We must dissect bad outcomes, identify bad judgment, and learn from these experiences. By doing so, we can garner the experience that shapes good judgment and provide optimal patient care.

12.4   Savor Your Victories

I keep all the thank-you notes from grateful patients in my second desk drawer. For mistakes, I have a mental file that replays on nights I can't sleep: the near misses, the missed diagnoses, the wrong decisions live there. The thank-you notes are locked in a drawer that I seldom open. The mistakes are never far from my mind.

It is human nature to remember your failures and forget your successes. An essential component of self-care is celebrating your victories—in fact, don't just celebrate them, savor them. Keep a mental file of the victories to sustain you when you feel uncertain and discouraged.

One of my favorite saves: I cared for a young transplant patient admitted after a routine angiogram which showed cardiac allograft vasculopathy. He underwent percutaneous coronary intervention and was set to be discharged the next day. Right before discharge, the resident called me because the patient had gone into atrial fibrillation with pauses.

I rushed to the bedside, calling the cardiothoracic surgery attending on call as I jogged up the stairs. The resident was surprised by my sense of urgency. Lacking experience, he considered this arrhythmia to be relatively benign—and he would have been right, if this were a non-transplant patient. However, atrial fibrillation with pauses can be a transplant emergency, a sentinel event that precedes imminent cardiovascular collapse.

The cardiothoracic surgeon and I arrived at the patient's bedside together. In the time it took me to race across the hospital, the patient had gone into cardiac arrest and was receiving cardiopulmonary resuscitation. Within what seemed like minutes, the cardiothoracic surgeon placed the patient on extracorporeal membrane oxygenation. Miraculously, the patient survived the arrest and years later, is thriving after a successful second transplant.

The cardiothoracic surgeon is the true hero of the story. However, my experience allowed me to recognize the imminent danger of the patient's arrhythmia. I was proud of myself: I efficiently alerted the cardiothoracic surgeon to expeditiously place the support that saved the patient's life. There are many losses in medicine that are out of our control; give yourself credit when it is due and savor your victories.

12.5 Find the Joy

When people ask me why I chose to become a heart transplant cardiologist, I explain that it's because I'm a drama queen. I am honored to watch patients as they are snatched from the jaws of death, transformed by the miracle of a donor heart. People think I'm joking, but I'm not. It's a rare and beautiful privilege to see something work that shouldn't. How is it that you can take someone's heart out, and put another heart in, and it beats? It's a miracle every time.

Even more incredible are the details that make each patient's story special. The mother with peripartum cardiomyopathy who received a heart transplant on Mother's Day. The veteran who fought in Iraq whose heart transplant anniversary is the Fourth of July. The proud Irish-American woman who handed out green shamrocks pins to everyone in the hospital and received a heart transplant on—you guessed it—Saint Patrick's Day. Don't take the small miracles for granted; cherish and celebrate these tiny joys.

I love to focus on how far patients have come: the middle-aged patient who underwent a heart transplant in her 20 s who asked me if it was safe to get Botox and fillers, and then blushed, self-consciously, because she never thought that she would live long enough to worry about wrinkles. I asked her to keep me posted on the cosmetic procedures she liked best since we were growing old together. Another incredible story: the heart transplant recipient who came to clinic on the 27th anniversary of his transplant with his daughter—who's 25. I love the moments in transplant clinic when the patients ask if it's okay to ride a roller coaster or scuba dive or paint their house (by themselves).

Heart transplantation is a specialty filled with miracles and tragedies. The joy of these tiny moments can create a raft of good memories to sustain you from the flood of tragedy. Regardless of your specialty, medicine is filled with these moments: find them, remember them, rejoice in them.

12.6   Final Thoughts

You will have moments of grief, fear, and doubt. You will question your abilities. When faced with these challenges, lean on trusted mentors and colleagues to talk you through. Judge yourself by your actions, which you can control, and not by the outcomes, which often you cannot.

Reference

Letter from Helen B. Taussig to Adrian Kantrowitz Alan Mason Chesney Medical Archives. Helen B. Taussig Collection 1968. https://profiles.nlm.nih.gov/101584941X156.

Chapter 13
What Covid-19 Has Taught Us (or Not)

The idea for this book started in the spring of 2019, well before the phrase "Covid-19" meant anything to anyone. It's hard to remember, but there was a time when no one had an involuntary shiver at the thought of crowded movie theaters or subways or touched their face before leaving the house to make sure they were wearing a mask. We did not think twice about hugging friends or sitting cheek-to-jowl in the hottest new restaurant, shouting over the table to be heard over the din of music and plates and cutlery.

I'm not an epidemiologist or infectious disease expert, and decidedly not an amateur armchair one either. But no one escaped the pall of Covid-19, which placed the world in a vise of existential dread. Covid-19 provided many lessons on the art and science of patient care. While none of these lessons are new and many are covered in earlier chapters, Covid-19 accelerated and heightened their importance.

13.1 The Myth of Zero Risk

When I recommend that a patient be evaluated for heart transplantation, I make sure to explain that while a heart transplant is a miracle and gift of life, it brings its own problems. There can be surgical complications, rejection, infection, and side effects of immunosuppression. The goal is to chart a course of minimal risk because there are no guarantees of zero risk. We choose the path that affords the greatest chance of optimal quality of life and survival—and that path is often transplantation. Words like odds and bet are appropriate because we are using the science of uncertainty and the art of probability to guide us. There is no such thing as zero risk; when making medical decisions, play the odds and always recognize that there will be a tradeoff.

Covid-19 is no different, though the decision-making played out on the world's stage rather than in a clinic exam room. Thanks to social media, we were privy to every angle of the argument for and against widespread, government-mandated lockdowns and school shutdowns that occurred almost without interruption between

© The Author(s), under exclusive license to Springer Nature Switzerland AG 2022   177
M. Kittleson, *Mastering the Art of Patient Care*,
https://doi.org/10.1007/978-3-031-20920-8_13

March 2020 and March 2021. There were strict restrictions around outdoor spaces like parks and playgrounds and beaches and outdoor dining.

There were benefits: flattening the curve to prevent hospitals from becoming overwhelmed, from repurposing operative rooms as intensive care units, from turning dermatology residents into intensivists. There were also risks: flattening the curve would not change the area under the curve; the spread of the virus could only be quelled by immunity to the virus (whether by infection or vaccination), not isolation from the virus, and isolation was not sustainable.

During the shutdown to flatten the curve, we accepted the risks to essential workers who couldn't stay home, like postal workers, grocery store employees, and everyone in health care, from physicians to nurses to the custodial staff. We acknowledged that humans as social creatures would still congregate, but perhaps that congregation would occur indoors, in secret, instead of in well-ventilated outdoor spaces. We accepted the risks to schoolchildren during school shutdowns, with potential risks ranging from a lack of structure to support from teachers and peers to education to socialization.

The choices we have made about Covid-19 are no different from the decisions we make every day for patients: we choose the path of lowest risk not zero risk. In patients with chronic pain, we do not titrate pain medication to zero pain. This is an unrealistic and often unattainable goal and the toxicity of the pain medication will exceed the benefit. Rather, we titrate pain medication to tolerable pain, balancing the risks of pain with the risks of over-administration of pain medication.

What is the level of tolerable Covid pain? I don't know the answer. Can it be zero? The first lesson we should learn from Covid is to keep an open mind. Consider all sides of the decision: what's the best-case scenario and worst-case scenario of each decision point, and which offers the best chance of success?

13.2 The Road to Bad Outcomes

In mid-March 2020, a longstanding patient called my office, asking for hydroxy-chloroquine to ward off COVID-19. His call came on the heels of a press conference touting the miracle of this wonder drug. I had managed his stable ischemic cardiomy-opathy for over a decade and in that time, he had called me only once, from Europe, when hospitalized with shortness of breath. A continent away, I could not titrate diuretic therapy or optimize afterload reduction. But I called him every day because he told me that my familiar voice on the phone was comfort enough. When he returned to Los Angeles, he hugged me tight, tears in his eyes, and I could feel the trust between us growing stronger.

After the presidential endorsement of hydroxychloroquine, I had braced myself for a flood of patient calls. Though I am a cardiologist, I had prepared a response based on evaluation of peer-reviewed publications, scientific statements, and internet anecdotes. I could have punted to his internist because that would have been easier than denying his request, but I did not. He trusted me, and I owed him an explanation for why I would not prescribe prophylactic hydroxychloroquine. Part of me wished I could prescribe hydroxychloroquine, to avoid his frustration and the threat of a negative patient review—but I didn't succumb.

I began with the theory: in vitro, hydroxychloroquine inhibits growth of SARS-CoV-2. I contrasted the theory with the practice: there was no evidence that hydroxychloroquine prevented COVID-19, reduced the severity of illness, or increased survival. I outlined the potential side effects and drug interactions. Finally, I appealed to his ethics: if I were to prescribe unnecessary hydroxychloroquine for him, then the supply might be compromised for patients with serious inflammatory conditions such as lupus or rheumatoid arthritis.

I expected chagrin; I was not prepared for his anger. He told me that "everyone" said hydroxychloroquine worked. How could I withhold this medical miracle? Since I would not give him hydroxychloroquine, he would investigate other sources. I could not stop thinking about our conversation that had gone so wrong. For ten years, he had arrived at his bi-annual appointments on time and never questioned my advice. When stranded in Europe, I was the physician he trusted enough to call. What had changed? He had weighed my medical expertise against that of the President and found me lacking. Did he really not trust me anymore?

I could not prescribe prophylactic hydroxychloroquine based on wishful thinking. As every student of clinical trials knows, the path to bad outcomes is paved with plausible surrogate endpoints. As discussed in Chap. 5, anyone who ever administered flecainide to suppress premature ventricular contractions (PVCs) after myocardial infarction (Echt et al 1991), post-menopausal hormonal therapy to improve lipid profiles (Manson et al 2003), or thiazoladinediones to reduce hemoglobin A1c in diabetic patients (Lipscombe et al 2007) has learned the dangers of surrogate endpoints. Reducing the burden of PVCs, the level of low-density lipoprotein cholesterol, and hemoglobin A1c are noble goals, yet medications to effect these changes result in arrhythmic death, coronary heart disease, and heart failure.

Then, all at once, I remembered how scared he was, in that Italian hospital years prior, and how my voice on the phone had been enough to comfort him. As scared as he was then, he was more so now. When we spoke, I had failed to address the emotion behind the question. He might have requested hydroxychloroquine, but what he needed was reassurance. He had asked for comfort and I had responded with science. As a different President, Teddy Roosevelt, said, "Nobody cares how much you know until they know how much you care." And this time, I had failed to convince him that I cared.

I reached out a few days later. I told him that while I could not prescribe prophylactic hydroxychloroquine, I understood why he wanted it. I validated his unspoken fear: as an older man with a cardiac condition, he was at risk of fatal respiratory failure from COVID-19. I expected that voicing his greatest fear might upset him more; instead, he was relieved that I did not minimize the danger.

I explained that while I understood his fear, I could not be swayed by it. As physicians, our decisions must be based on available evidence, not on hope or panic. What if, after I declined to prescribe hydroxychloroquine, he died of COVID-19, and, months later, hydroxychloroquine was proven effective as prophylaxis? On the other hand, what if I gave in and prescribed hydroxychloroquine, he took it for the sniffles, and suffered fatal polymorphic ventricular tachycardia? The former would be tragic but the latter would be unforgiveable.

I did not expect to change his mind, and I was not surprised when he called me a week later to let me know that he had obtained a stash of hydroxychloroquine from "another source." The tension between anecdotes and data, between giving a patient what they want versus what they need, has always threatened to break the trust between patients and physicians. COVID-19 simply heightens these tensions. With the risk of imminent death and the lure of unproven wonder drugs, reason can fall prey to emotion. But there was a small silver lining: he promised that he would not take any hydroxychloroquine without contacting me first, and I believed him.

He ended our call by asking, "Are we okay?" He too sought to repair our fractured trust. I had science on my side, but he had the fear of death on his; we could disagree on the best way to remain safe in the pandemic and still trust each other. The fear and uncertainty of COVID-19 may strain the patient-physician bond, but it need not break it. Patients need to know that we, as physicians, will not abandon them if we disagree. When the pandemic ends, our trust will be stronger for it.

This story is about hydroxychloroquine, but it could just as easily apply to any of the fads that have played out during the Covid pandemic. It's not "how can it [hydroxychloroquine, azithromycin, vitamin D, famotidine, fluvoxamine, ivermectin, anticoagulation, holding ACE inhibitors] hurt?" Rather, it's "how can it harm?" It may feel like emotion and desperation have replaced logic and science. Put logic and science first. Just because you can do something, does not mean you should. While it is harder to do nothing or to say no, have the courage of your convictions.

13.3   Disagreement and Covid

The strategies outlined in Chap. 9 will help you navigate the medical, emotional, and political quagmire of the Covid vaccine. Avoid emotional appeals as you incorporate medical facts with the patient's perspective. Such appeals can turn antagonistic, alienating the patient and moving you farther away from the goal of optimal patient care. When the issue at hand impacts only the patient, it is easier to separate fact from emotion. When the issue at hand impacts society on a larger scale, such as disagreement over the benefits of the Covid vaccine, it will be much harder to avoid an emotional appeal.

I care for a medically vulnerable population of heart transplant recipients at high risk of death from Covid. Many of these patients have trusted me to guide them through the often risky, painful, and even investigational interventions on the road to transplantation. Yet, when faced with my recommendation that they protect themselves from Covid by vaccination, some patients decline. The reasons range from, "I need more research," to "I won't get Covid anyway" to "You told me I can't take ibuprofen but a vaccine is okay?".

When faced with reasons like these, do your best to counter the mistrust in the science, the misplaced optimism, and the illogical connections. For my heart transplant patients, I explain the risks of Covid infection to them: in large series of heart transplant recipients who contract Covid, about two-thirds of patients require hospitalization and 15% die (Genuardi et al 2021). I contrast these risks with those of the vaccine: a sore arm and some flu-like symptoms. I try to approach every question with respect, whether it be about the benefits of hydroxychloroquine or the risks of sterility from the vaccine. I conclude by emphasizing our shared goal: to keep them safe and healthy. When you explain the risks of Covid versus the risks of the vaccine to your patients, try to do so gently, and always end with, "I care about you and need to explain my medical recommendations to keep you safe and healthy. I understand that you will ultimately make the decision you feel is right."

Because their lives hang in the balance, I want to shake sense into my patients, even force them to agree with me. Instead, play the long game. When a patient declines my recommendation and eschews vaccination, a decision that may hurt them and those around them, I feel hurt and insulted. Still, I end the conversation with respect and acceptance. The end of the conversation is not the end of the discussion. Preserve the patient-physician relationship. Look ahead to the other opportunities you will have to explain, convince, and hopefully change their minds.

The stakes are higher in a discussion about vaccination, and not just the medical stakes of protecting the patient and society from Covid. The stakes of maintaining trust and maintaining the patient-physician bond are higher too. Despite your strong emotions, focus on the medical facts, avoid engaging in counterproductive emotional arguments, and end with acceptance.

13.4   Final Thoughts

Covid is a microcosm of all that is challenging and rewarding in medicine. In the crucible of fear and mistrust, we learned to continue to be guided by science as we balanced risks, critically evaluated the surrogate endpoints of clinical trials, and prioritized the patient-physician relationship when threatened by disagreement. When in doubt, remember the lessons of the Golden Rule of medicine—don't do anything to a patient unless it will help them feel better and/or live longer—and have the courage to say no if what the patient thinks they want will not help.

References

Echt DS, Liebson PR, Mitchell LB, et al. Mortality and morbidity in patients receiving encainide, flecainide, or placebo. N Engl J Med. 1991;324:781–8.
Genuardi MV, Moss N, Najjar SS, et al. Coronavirus disease 2019 in heart transplant recipients: risk factors, immunosuppression, and outcomes. J Heart Lung Transplant. 2021;40:926–35.

Lipscombe LL, Gomes T, Lévesque LE, Hux JE, Juurlink DN, Alter DA. Thiazolidinediones and cardiovascular outcomes in older patients with diabetes. JAMA. 2007;298:2634–43.

Manson JE, Hsia J, Johnson KC, et al. Estrogen plus progestin and the risk of coronary heart disease. N Engl J Med. 2003;349:523–34.

Afterword: The Joy of Medicine

There will be highs and lows in your career. There will be times when you are grateful for the privilege of being a physician and times when you question whether it is the right career for you. The rigor of training includes a million tiny paper cuts to your confidence: you are never certain of the right approach, you are always at the starting line of the learning curve, you have to rely on others for approval, and you need this approval for advancement.

Medicine will take up much of your life. You will spend years honing your craft. The stress and uncertainty will be an additional emotional drain. Yet, you will build the stamina to endure the stress and uncertainty for years on end. You will maintain that stamina and the return on investment is enormous. You will have the privilege of knowing how the body works and the ability to use this scientific expertise to help people feel better and live longer. You will be given intimate glimpses into the lives of your patients and see them at their best and, unfortunately, also at their worst. You will have a hand in orchestrating their greatest joys and comforting them through their greatest tragedies. You will be compassionate but not overly emotional, experienced but not complacent, and calm but never cold. You will learn when to be cautious but not fearful and bold but not reckless.

I have had hard days in medicine. I remember the exhaustion of overnight call in the intensive care unit, collapsing in my bed, intending to take a 20-min afternoon nap and waking up 13 h later, disoriented and panicked. I had missed dinner with friends, had forgotten to put the laundry in the dryer—but at least I had caught up on much-needed sleep.

I have had harder days in medicine. I remember the uncertainty of the early days: did I have the talent or expertise to provide optimal patient care? There were days when my fellow trainees seemed to know every answer at morning report, and I knew none. There were moments when I knew I was failing in my attempt to garner a patient's trust, and I did not know how to salvage the conversation. There were times when patients suffered terrible outcomes, and I wondered if my lack of talent or expertise contributed to the tragedies.

M. Kittleson, *Mastering the Art of Patient Care*,
https://doi.org/10.1007/978-3-031-20920-8

The exhaustion and uncertainty of medical training can be overwhelming—and it doesn't end with training. The press is rife with stories of burnout in healthcare workers. What is the source of burnout? Is it the hard work itself or, rather, is it the uncertainty of not knowing if your hard work is serving an important purpose? Without a sense of purpose, you lose sight of medicine as a hallowed tradition and a coveted vocation. How do you maintain the sense of purpose that is a key ingredient in the joy of medicine? In a word: connection. A sense of purpose is forged through connection: mentors and trusted colleagues will support and sustain you through moments of exhaustion and uncertainty.

For decades now, my mentors and trusted colleagues have given me a safe space to vent and recharge and, along with my patients, have sustained my sense of purpose in medicine. Because of their encouragement, I could awaken from a 13-h hibernation in the early days ready to return to the hospital and keep returning, over decades, to experience the joy of medicine. They motivated me to learn more rather than become discouraged that I did not know enough. They gave me courage to dissect bad outcomes and apply the lessons to improve the care of future patients. I recognized that all my mentors had a system. I knew I needed one too, so I incorporated their styles and practices to create my own.

My patients, mentors, and trusted colleagues have provided the valuable experience that inspired the systems and concrete action plans in this book. These systems can be one of the tools you use to ease the unique and overwhelming challenges of medical school and beyond. However, while these systems may set you on the right path, the connections you make with patients, mentors, and trusted colleagues will maintain your true course. Even better, as you mentor others, you will foster new connections to reignite the joy of medicine. Like your family at home, your work family will grow for generations and will flourish with care and consideration. Nurturing strong work relationships is essential to providing optimal patient care.

Let this book be the opening statements, not the concluding remarks, of an ongoing conversation in medicine. Let us continue to discuss our experience and and share wisdom. In doing so, we will maintain the joy of medicine and make a difference in patient's lives.